**Tutorials for
Junior Students
of Surgery**

Tutorials for Junior Students of Surgery

Graham L Hill MD, CHM, FRACS, FRCS, FACS
Professor and Chairman, Department of Surgery, University of Auckland School of Medicine, Auckland, New Zealand

Andrew G Hill MB, CHB
House Surgeon, Auckland Hospital, Auckland, New Zealand

Churchill Livingstone
EDINBURGH, LONDON, MELBOURNE AND NEW YORK 1990

CHURCHILL LIVINGSTONE
Medical Division of Longman Group UK Limited

Distributed in the United States of America by
Churchill Livingstone Inc., 1560 Broadway, New York,
N.Y. 10036, and by associated companies, branches and
representatives throughout the world.

© Graham L Hill 1989

All rights reserved; no part of this publication may be
reproduced, stored in a retrieval system, or transmitted in any
form or by any means, electronic, mechanical, photocopying,
recording or otherwise, without either the prior written
permission of the Publishers (Churchill Livingstone,
Robert Stevenson House, 1-3 Baxter's Place, Leith Walk,
Edinburgh EH1 3AF) or a licence permitting restricted copying
in the United Kingdom issued by the Copyright Licensing
Agency Ltd, 33-34 Alfred Place, London WC1E 7DP.

First published 1989
Churchill Livingstone edition 1990

ISBN 0-443-04449-X

Printed in Great Britain by
Butler & Tanner Ltd, Frome and London

PREFACE

Our principal aim in producing "Tutorials for Junior Students of Surgery" was to provide a core of material that needs to be known by our students by the end of their first 'surgical run'. These tutorials are simply an introduction to surgical disease and will help to make clinical work more meaningful and discussion with teachers more substantial. They are not an alternative to standard accounts in textbooks but are designed to give an overview and perspective which is complimentary to the more comprehensive descriptions contained in them.

Indeed, it is anticipated that the student will read these tutorials alongside the prescribed text book fleshing out the material contained here and producing a more personal 'text' for him or her self.

We would like to thank the General Surgeons within the Department of Surgery at Auckland Medical School who helped with the project. Mr Ian Civil (Trauma, Peripheral Vascular Disease), Mr Tom Morris (Diseases of the Venous System), and Associate Professor Ronald Kay (Carcinoma of the Breast) provided tutorials and Associate Professor James Shaw and Mr John Collins gave valuable advice. Fourth year students Louise Finnel, Tony Scott and Philip Hill gave useful input, and Douglas Hill and Mrs Bartha Hill worked hard on many aspects of production. The whole enterprise was made possible by a generous grant from Baxter Healthcare Limited.

G L H
A G H

CONTENTS

1	Preparing the Patient for Surgery	1
2	Perioperative Care	6
3	Metabolic Care of the Surgical Patient	12
4	The Acute Abdomen	24
5	Surgical (Obstructive) Jaundice	35
6	Haematemesis, Melaena and Peptic Ulcer Disease	44
7	Bleeding from the Anus, Rectum and Colon	51
8	Swellings of the Thyroid Gland (Goitre) and other Swellings of the Head and Neck	60
9	Carcinoma of the Breast	67
10	Swellings of the Groin	76
11	Trauma	82
12	Peripheral Vascular Disease	89
13	Diseases of the Venous System	97
14	Common Skin Malignancies	106
Index		111

Tutorial 1

Preparing the Patient for Surgery

There are not many life events more important to a patient than a major operation. The surgeon's first contact with the patient is crucial. He will seek to gain the patient's confidence and reassure him/her that help is available. There are data which suggest that a properly counselled patient requires less post operative pain relief and spends less time in hospital. Once the diagnosis has been made and the risks of surgery have been properly assessed the surgeon will describe the proposed procedure to the patient, its chances of success, its risks and any alternatives. This is done in a way the patient can understand, with sympathy and understanding. In all this, the surgeon - general practitioner interaction is of vital importance. Both before and after the operation the lion's share of the overall care of the patient and his family is taken by the general practitioner. This is why the general practitioner writes an initial referral letter explaining the patient's problem and this is why the surgeon writes back giving his opinion and later describing the operative findings and the postoperative recovery and likely prognosis.

PREOPERATIVE EVALUATION

One or two weeks before admission to hospital the patient attends an outpatient assessment clinic where a thorough history is taken, a full physical examination is undertaken and a number of investigations are arranged. In this way, organic, physiological, biochemical or psychiatric disturbances can be evaluated and possible anaesthetic or surgical difficulties are anticipated. The *history* entails asking questions about respiratory disease and smoking, cardiac and vascular disease including deep vein thrombosis, and other medical disorders including bleeding diathesis, hypertension and diabetes. Current medications and drug allergies are asked about as are previous anaesthetic experiences.

The *physical examination* is a complete one evaluating all systems and *investigations* routinely include blood grouping and antibody screen, haemoglobin and a chest radiograph. An electrocardiogram should be carried out in all patients over 50 years and those with cardiac disease or hypertension. Urea and electrolyte estimation are performed in all patients undergoing major surgery, in patients on diuretics, suspected renal impairment or patients on intravenous fluid therapy. Pulmonary function tests, sputum culture and blood gas analysis are reserved for patients with respiratory disease and clotting factor studies are performed in all patients with haemorrhagic disease or jaundice.

PATIENTS AT INCREASED RISK

Elderly Patients

Patients over the age of 70 years have a 3-4 times increased incidence of major complications and death after surgery. Physiological adaptation to major surgery is impaired in elderly subjects. They react less well to haemorrhage, fluid shifts, anoxia, sepsis and medications. For these reasons very major procedures are undertaken with caution in the elderly. During the operative procedure great care is taken in matching fluid requirements to losses, to ensuring full oxygenation, and in prescribing medications. Postoperatively opiates are given in small doses if at all.

Obese Patients

Obese patients provide both the anaesthetist and the surgeon with a number of special problems. Venous access and establishment of an airway can be very difficult in very obese patients. All operations are more difficult and dangerous when fat stores are large and postoperatively there is an increased risk of cardiovascular death, deep vein thrombosis, wound and chest infections.

Malnourished Patients

It is generally believed that patients with major weight loss have an increased morbidity and mortality after surgery. This is not entirely true, however, for it has now been established that physiological impairment must be present as well as weight loss. In these circumstances the risk of postoperative complications is 2-3 times higher and the incidence of postoperative sepsis is increased. Thus if a patient has a recent weight loss of more than 15% of his well weight and is noted on physical examination to have a markedly impaired grip strength and/or is unable to blow over a strip of paper held 10 cm from his mouth then preoperative nutritional replenishment is indicated. Usually 5-7 days of enteral or parenteral nutrition is all that is required to improve these impairments.

Hypoalbuminaemic Patients

Hypoalbuminaemia (plasma albumin < 35 g/l) is a major risk factor for postoperative complications. It usually indicates overt or occult sepsis and for this reason most surgeons will, if possible, avoid very major surgery in such patients.

Diabetic Patients

Hypoglycaemia, a potentially fatal occurrence, may occur in diabetic patients while under anaesthesia. This is prevented by giving an infusion of insulin and dextrose during anaesthesia and doing frequent blood sugar estimations.

Patients with Pulmonary Dysfunction

Patients with respiratory disease have an increased risk of pneumonia and wound disruption postoperatively. Cessation of smoking, bronchodilators, chest physiotherapy and postural drainage may decrease these risks.

Patients with Cardiovascular Disease

It will be shown in the next tutorial that a recent myocardial infarction has a profound influence on postoperative recovery.

Patients with valvular disease may develop subacute bacterial endocarditis postoperatively and for this reason prophylactic antibiotics are prescribed.

PREOPERATIVE PREPARATION

There are a number of important procedures the patient needs to undergo during the twelve hour period prior to surgery:

Preparation of the Gastro Intestinal Tract

Solid food is omitted for 12 hours preoperatively and fluids for at least 6 hours. If the operation is on the large bowel, that will be cleaned by the patient drinking Golytely. This consists of a balanced crystalloid solution of Polyethylene Glycol. About 2 l of this orange flavoured solution achieves very satisfactory mechanical cleansing of the bowel.

Prophylactic Antibiotics

Whenever the surgeon anticipates that the gastrointestinal tract will be opened at any stage of the operation he will prescribe broad spectrum antibiotics before operation and during the first post operative day to reduce the risk of wound infection. Prophylactic antibiotics are timed so that therapeutic levels are achieved in the blood at the time of surgery.

Prophylaxis against Deep Vein Thrombosis (D.V.T.)

The risk of D.V.T. in patients undergoing surgical treatment is influenced by a number of factors which include age, nature and extent of the operation, presence of varicose veins, malignant disease, obesity, cardiac disease and a history of previous D.V.T. or pulmonary embolism. Since the risk is very low in patients under the age of 40 years undergoing short operations, specific prophylaxis is not used but for all other patients graduated compression stockings, or low dose heparin, or external pneumatic compression either singly or in combination are used. The graduated compression stockings are worn throughout the hospital stay. Low dose heparin is administered 2 hours before the operation and then every 12 hours until the patient is up and about around the ward. External pneumatic compression is performed by encasing the patient's leg in an envelope of plastic material, and rhythmically allowing the pressure to squeeze the calf muscles and encourage venous return. This is done to prevent stasis during the operation itself.

Preparation of the Skin

Hair from the operative site is removed by clipping and the area is washed thoroughly with soap and water.

Preparation for Anaesthesia

A short time before going to the operation suite many patients are given sedatives to reduce fear and stress. Anticholinergic agents may also be given to reduce the amount of saliva and bronchial secretions produced in response to the anaesthetist's endo-tracheal tube.

FURTHER READING FOR INTEREST

Mainland, J.F., Weeks, A.M. (1988): Minimum Requirements for Anaesthesia with respect to checking the Patient, Medical Tests, Work-up. Anaesthetic Intens. Care $\underline{16}$: 22-24

FURTHER READING FOR FINALS

Way, L.W. : Current Surgical Diagnosis and Treatment. 5th Edition, 1988. Appleton and Lange . pp 6-14 , 67, 107.

NOTES

Tutorial 2

Perioperative Care

Skilled care does not stop when the patient leaves the operating theatre door. In fact, for the trainee intern and housesurgeon, this is where it really begins. The careful work of the anaesthetist and the surgeon in the operating theatre must continue on to the ward if it is to be of lasting benefit. An understanding of the physiological and metabolic effects of surgery is therefore important.

PHYSIOLOGICAL EFFECTS OF SURGERY

The operation itself causes a number of physiological effects. Nearly every aspect of respiratory function is impaired by general anaesthesia. Ventilation, lung perfusion, gas exchange, mucus clearance and the cough reflex are all affected. The entire coagulation cascade culminates in a burst of thrombin activity. There may be major losses of body heat. Extracellular fluid is sequestered around the dissection site (about 1 litre for every 2 hours of operating time) and red cells and plasma are lost. The anaesthetist monitors and controls these physiological effects by the proper choice of anaesthetic agents, controlled ventilation techniques, the use of warming apparatus, and replacement of extracellular fluid, plasma and red cells.

METABOLIC EFFECTS OF SURGERY

The operation also causes a number of important metabolic effects. There is an increase in protein catabolism, a relative decrease in protein anabolism and an alteration in glucose metabolism. Increased amounts of nitrogen, potassium, zinc, magnesium and calcium are excreted in the urine while sodium and water are retained. The origin of the increased nitrogen loss in the urine (as well as potassium, magnesium and zinc) is muscle. This metabolic response to the operation is initiated by fear and apprehension and particularly by afferent impulses from the site of surgery. Rapid changes in circulating blood volume as well as the release of peptides from the damaged tissues also are important factors. These metabolic effects are mediated by circulating hormones which are increased as a result of operative trauma. Cortisol, adrenaline, noradrenaline, aldosterone, ADH, ACTH, and growth hormone are all increased. There is a reversal of the normal glucagon/insulin ratio as well. The observation that increased hormone levels in the blood after surgery are related to fear, anxiety, tissue damage and hypovolaemia emphasize the importance of the careful preparation of the patient prior to operation, the gentle handling of tissues by the surgeon and the maintenance of an adequate circulating blood volume as prime objectives of peri-operative care.

EARLY POST OPERATIVE COURSE

Management

As soon as the operation is over, attention is paid to waking the patient up, pain relief and fluid balance. He or she is taken to the recovery room and is there monitored for some time by skilled anaesthetic and nursing staff. When the patient is breathing spontaneously and is stable, he/she is taken to the ward where the surgical team takes over management. Pain relief is achieved in a number of ways which include the continuous use of opiate analgesia delivered intravenously using a pain pump, the intermittent intramuscular injection of opiates or the interpleural injection of local anaesthetic.

The next problem facing the housesurgeon is that of fluid balance. The general surgical patient will have an intravenous drip in place and may have a nasogastric tube as well to prevent gastric dilatation as stomach (and colonic) motility is discoordinate and slow. The catabolic state lasts for approximately 24 - 48 hours and results in sodium and water retention and the release of intracellular nitrogen and potassium to the extracellular fluid. It is for this reason that in the first 24 hours postoperatively no potassium is added to *maintenance* intravenous solutions which should provide 2 litres of water and 60 mmols of sodium. If urine volume does not reach 30-40 mls per hour, then plasma substitutes(e.g. Stable Plasma Protein Solution-SPPS) and extracellular fluid substitutes (e.g. Plasmalyte) are given to restore vascular and interstitial fluid volume respectively. By the next day the situation is usually stable and a simple maintenance regimen of 2500 mls water, 75 mmol sodium, and 50 mmol potassium is all that is required until the patient is able to take fluid orally. If difficulties are anticipated with fluid balance then an indwelling urinary catheter is inserted with or without a central line for measurement of the central venous pressure. Very ill patients with organ failure will be admitted to the department of critical care where they can be mechanically ventilated and a much more precise monitoring of fluid balance be obtained.

Difficulties That May Be Encountered

There are a number of problems which may develop in the first 24 hours postoperatively. The commonest are:

Bleeding

Careful monitoring of the pulse (increased rate but less volume) and blood pressure (progressive fall) may suggest continuing blood loss. If this does not respond to moderate replacement with resuspended red cells and S.P.P.S., then continuing bleeding is a possibility and the surgeon will be called to decide the proper course of action. A special case is thyroidectomy. If bleeding occurs into the neck after this operation the larynx may be compressed resulting in respiratory embarrassment. Urgent evacuation of the blood is required.

Urinary Retention

This commonly occurs in elderly men and is caused by a combination of bladder neck obstruction, lying in bed and abdominal pain preventing development of sufficient intraabdominal pressure to initiate micturition. Some operations such as herniorrhaphy and haemorrhoidectomy are particularly associated with urinary retention.
Retention is suspected in any restless patient who has not passed urine 6 hours after surgery. The diagnosis is made by palpation of the swollen tender bladder. Treatment is by insertion of a urinary catheter under sterile conditions.

Fever

The commonest cause of early postoperative fever greater than 38°C is atelectasis -alveoli which are closed in all phases of tidal respiration. It is predisposed to by chest pain or abdominal pain restricting free breathing and coughing. The cause is either bronchial obstruction by mucus or inadequate ventilation of alveoli; the distal air is absorbed, and the airways collapse. Intrapulmonary shunting occurs and this results in hypoxia which stimulates chemoreceptors producing reflex tachpnoea and hyperpnoea. Treatment is physiotherapy (deep breathing and coughing exercises) oxygen, adequate pain relief and satisfactory hydration so as to decrease the tenacity of the mucus.

LATER POSTOPERATIVE COURSE (DAYS 3-7)

Management

The metabolic response to the operation is now over and the patient begins to take an interest in his/her appearance and surroundings. As soon as flatus is passed the nasogastric tube can be removed and sips of water commenced. When the bowels are moving, food can be eaten. By the end of the first week the patient is eating small meals and is up and about around the ward. Wound clips or sutures are removed about this time.

Difficulties that may be encountered

Pneumonia

This occurs in about 15% of patients after major surgery. If atelectasis is not dealt with adequately as soon as it is recognized then pneumonia may result. In the younger patient it is not difficult to make the diagnosis but it may be more difficult in the elderly patient. Whenever pneumonia is suspected a physical examination (high fever, high pulse, increased respiratory rate with bronchial breathing) and a chest X ray are performed. Treatment is pain relief, physiotherapy, and the use of appropriate antibiotics and oxygen.

Wound Complications

Infection
Most wound infections are usually caused by endogenous rather than exogenous bacterial contamination. For this reason the surgeon takes care to reduce contamination which occurs when a viscus is opened or an abscess is drained. He will appose the wound edges accurately and without tension using staples, skin tapes or sutures. It is possible for bacteria to migrate into a wound for two or three days after surgery and for this reason the wound is sealed with a plastic dressing which is left undisturbed for 3-4 days. In 5-10% of patients, discharge of pus or infected material from the wound (i.e. wound infection) may occur towards the end of the first post operative week. Treatment involves removal of sutures, drainage of the pus and packing of the gaping wound.

Dehiscence
Partial or total disruption of any or all layers of the operative wound occurs in about 2% of abdominal surgical procedures. Evisceration is when all layers of the abdominal wall are ruptured and the viscera protrude through it. Leakage of serous fluid from an abdominal wound after 4-5 days may be an impending sign of wound dehiscence. Wound evisceration with the sudden appearance of bowel loops is a frightening event. The patient is returned to the operating room immediately and the wound is resutured.

Myocardial Infarction (M.I.)

The main risk of a myocardial infarction is between 3 and 5 days postoperatively.

Up to 50% of postoperative MIs occur silently and they manifest themselves as continuous hypo or hypertension, arrythmias or congestive heartfailure. Up to 60% of postoperative MIs result in death. The risk of postoperative MI in patients with no previous cardiac history is 0.5 %. The risk increases from 6%, in patients who have had an MI more than 6 months prior to operation, to 30% if infarction has occurred within 3 months of operation.

Deep Venous Thrombosis(DVT) and Pulmonary Embolus (PE)

Calf vein thrombosis (D.V.T.) occurs in 10-15% of patients undergoing major surgery. It is secondary to hypercoagulability of the blood and immobility of the calf muscle pumps during anaesthesia. Calf vein thrombosis may predispose to venous insuffiency in later life but its main danger is that it may extend proximally into the ilio-femoral veins and release a pulmonary embolus. Certain patients are at high risk - the elderly,the obese, patients with cancer and those with chronic venous insufficiency. In such patients the precautions discussed in Tutorial 1 are taken to reduce these risks. Clinically, DVT is suspected when physical examination reveals local calf distension, tenderness, oedema, discoloration, pain and the patient has a fever. Most often, though,clinical diagnosis alone is unreliable and the diagnosis is made by venography.Treatment is at first intravenous heparin and later oral anticoagulants.

Clinical diagnosis of PE depends to a large extent on the degree of vascular obstruction. Pleural pain and haemoptysis more often reflect submassive embolism whereas syncope indicates masive embolism. Only 15% of patients develop classic ECG changes. The diagnosis is best made by a radio-isotope perfusion lung scan. Radio-isotope labelled particles are injected intravenously; these particles lodge in the pre-capillary arterioles and capillaries in the lung, and their distribution reflects pulmonary blood flow. If there is pulmonary vascular obstruction, an underperfused area of lung scan can be detected by a gamma camera. A pulmonary angiogram is the definitive method for diagnosis of a pulmonary embolus. Treatment is at first intravenous heparin and later oral anticoagulants.

FURTHER READING FOR INTEREST

Bonica, J.J. (1982): Postoperative Pain (2 Parts); Contemporary Surgery 20, 83,119

FURTHER READING FOR FINALS

Way, L.W., Current Surgical Diagnosis and Treatment; 8th Edition, 1988
    Appleton and Lange, Pp 23-39

NOTES

Tutorial 3

Metabolic Care of the Surgical Patient

FLUID AND ELECTROLYTE THERAPY

Most surgical illness and operative intervention alter the balance and distribution of body water and electrolytes. A good understanding of the metabolism of salt, water and electrolytes is necessary for you to grasp the principles of pre and post operative care. In this section some basic concepts of surgical physiology will first be outlined before discussing some common changes in body fluids that occur in surgical illness and how each of them may be treated.

Surgical Physiology

Body Composition

The body mass is best thought of as being composed of the fat mass and the fat free or lean body mass. The latter comprises water (ECF and ICF), protein, minerals and glycogen (Figure 1)

Tissue	Mass
Fat	14kg
ECF	19L
ICF	23L
Protein	11kg
Minerals	2kg
Glycogen	1kg

Figure 1 Body composition of a normal 70 Kg male

Fat - contains no water and is therefore not involved in fluid and electrolyte physiology. It comprises a greater proportion of body weight in females and increases in both sexes with age. It provides the major energy source for surgical patients who are not eating or receiving nutritional support.

ECF - extra cellular fluid - contains sodium at 140 mmols per litre and potassium at 4 mmols per litre. It comprises plasma, interstitial fluid, connective tissue water and third space fluids

such as gastrointestinal tract water and intraocular fluid.
ICF - intracellular fluid - contains sodium at 10 mmols per litre and potassium at 150 mmols per litre. Extra cellular potassium is therefore but a tiny fraction of the total body content. In a fit young man with 19 L of E.C.F. only 70 mmol (out of a total body content of 3500 mmol) is outside cells. The total plasma potassium may vary from as little as 7 mmol in a small woman to 21 mmol in a large man.
Protein - Fifty five percent of the protein in the body is inside cells. This is the "engine of the body" where all metabolic processes take place. The other 45% forms the supporting structures of the body and is not involved in metabolic processes.
Minerals - mostly bone calcium and magnesium
Glycogen - It is in the liver and muscle and provides an energy store in short term starvation and in emergencies.

The distribution of Body Water in a 70 Kg Adult is shown in Figure 2 - intravenous fluids are distributed through these compartments within 2 hours of administration.

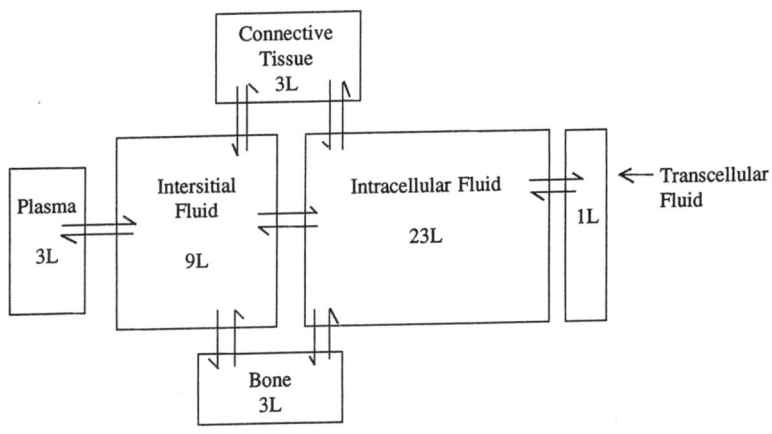

Figure 2   The Extracellular and Intracellular Water Compartments of the Body

If tritiated water is injected intravenously it is distributed throughout these compartments within 2 hours. Transcellular fluid is not metabolically available

Whole Body Osmolality

The body behaves as an osmometer, acting to keep the osmolality of all body fluids the same. The differences in ionic concentrations between the intracellular and extracellular compartments are due to the selective permeability of the cell membrane. Although water freely diffuses through this semi-permeable membrane the passage of sodium and its salts into the cell is retarded while that of potassium and its salts is promoted. This ability of water to diffuse freely across the cell membrane means that the osmolality of all body compartments is identical.

e.g. In surgical illness a common problem is hyponatraemia. Since sodium is the major cation in the E.C.F. this means that there is a decrease in effective osmotic pressure in the extracellular water resulting in diffusion of water into cells. This occurs also in nervous tissue and is one reason why patients with hyponatraemia get headaches.

Some Basic Facts Concerning Fluid and Electrolyte Balance

TABLE 1

24 Hour Average Intake and Output of Water in a 70 Kg Adult

	Intake		Output
Oral Liquids	1300 ml	Urine	1500 ml
Water in Food	900 ml	Stool	200 ml
Water of Oxidation	300 ml	Lungs	300 ml
		Skin	500 ml
	2500 ml		2500 ml

Note
The average subject requires 2500 mls of water per day.

TABLE 2

24 Hour Average Intake and Output of Sodium in a 70 Kg Adult

Intake	Output	
Diet 50-150 mmol/day	Urine	10-120 mmol/day
	Stool	0-20 mmol/day
	Skin	10-60 mmol/day

Note
The average subject requires about 75 mmol of sodium per day

Composition of Gastrointestinal Secretions

TABLE 3

	Volume (ml)	Na+ (mmol/l)	K+ (mmol/l)	Cl- (mmol/l)	HCO-3 (mmol/l)
Gastric Juice	1000	100	15	120	0
Pancreatic Fistula	700	140	5	75	120
Biliary Fistula	500	145	5	90	40
Jejunostomy	2000-3000	110	5	90	30
Ileostomy	500	115	8	45	30
Diarrhoeal Stools	500-15000	120	10	90	45

Note
The high concentration of chloride and the absence of bicarbonate in gastric juice. All the other secretions are for all practical purposes similar with the exception of pancreatic juice which is high in bicarbonate.

Common Fluid and Electrolyte Changes in Surgery

Volume Deficit (Surgical Dehydration, E.C.F. Depletion)

In surgical patients dehydration is not dehydration - it is "salt depletion". This statement emphasizes that E.C.F. depletion is the commonest fluid and electrolyte disorder encountered in surgical patients. On the other hand pure water deficit is very uncommon in surgical practice. Volume deficit results from *intestinal obstruction, vomiting, excessive diarrhoea, severe trauma, major surgery, extensive dissection, fluid loss* from *enterocutaneous fistulas, extensive burns, sepsis* and *shock*. The amount of E.C.F lost can be very large (Table 4) and is derived from the compartment with the greatest reserve (interstitial fluid) with initial protection of the circulating plasma volume. With a moderate deficit, therefore, E.C.F. depletion affects mainly the interstitial fluid compartment leading to loss of tissue turgor, dry tongue and thirst. As the capacity of the interstitial compartment diminishes, changes in circulating plasma volume occur with compensatory tachycardia and vasoconstriction. In severe depletion shock occurs.

The Signs and Symptoms of Surgical Dehydration are shown in Table 4

TABLE 4

Deficit	Mild (1-2 L ECF)	Moderate (2-4 L ECF)	Severe (5-9 L ECF)
Symptoms	Gives history of recent loss of ECF	Apathy, Anorexia Tachycardia Collapsed veins	Stupor or Coma Ileus
Signs	Usually no signs	Decreased Tissue turgor Dry tongue	Pale, Hypotensive Cold Extremities Absent Pulses Decreased Tissue turgor Sunken eyes

The deficits have been worked out for a normal 70 Kg male. When calculating the E.C.F. deficit for an individual adjustments should be made for the patient's body weight and degree of obesity. Remember, the more fat, the less lean. In other words, for 2 patients of equal weight the fatter patient has less fluid and electrolyte requirements.

For treatment the calculated deficit of E.C.F. is replaced by the intravenous administration of a fluid which resembles E.C.F., i.e. Normal Saline or Plasmalyte.

Hyponatraemia

This is the commonest disorder of electrolyte concentration in surgery and is due to a relative excess of water (free water). It is seen most often in postoperative patients who are having salt rich losses replaced with salt poor fluids.

Treatment is by water restriction and cautious replacement of calculated sodium requirements.

Hypokalaemia

A fall in 1 mmol of plasma potassium concentration in a 70 Kg subject indicates a 100-200 mmol deficit of total body potassium. Hypokalaemia in surgical patients most commonly occurs in patients with excessive gastrointestinal losses of sodium. As a consequence there is renal conservation of sodium with increased urinary excretion of potassium. Since ECF potassium is such a small proportion of the total body store of potassium it must be replaced very cautiously (no more than 15 mmol/hour).

Metabolic Alkalosis

This is a common disorder in surgical patients who have been vomiting or subjected to prolonged nasogastric suction. The basic mechanism is not only loss of fluid with high chloride and hydrogen ion concentration but volume loss as well which the kidney deals with by conserving sodium. With this avid salt conserving mechanism potassium and hydrogen ions are excreted in the urine in increasing quantities resulting in uncompensated alkalosis and hypokalaemia. The end result is *hypokalaemic, hypochloraemic, metabolic alkalosis* with a paradoxically acid urine. Treatment for this disorder is volume repletion with normal saline. Potassium supplementation is provided once an adequate urine output has been achieved.

Metabolic Acidosis

The commonest cause in surgical patients is acute circulatory failure causing tissue hypoxia and accumulation of lactic acid. The treatment of metabolic acidosis should be directed towards correction of the underlying disorder.

Other Disorders

Respiratory Acidosis occurs when respiration is inadequate and may be seen in postoperative patients who cannot breathe properly because of pain. *Respiratory alkalosis* is seen in hyperventilating patients and may be encountered in very anxious surgical patients. This is manifested as paraesthesiae in the fingers and lips and occasionally as carpopedal spasm.

Intravenous Solutions

There are a multitude of solutions available for the therapy of fluid and electrolyte disorders but in practice only four are needed. These four solutions are based on two simple solutions: "Normal Saline" and molar potassium chloride. Normal saline can be made by adding one teaspoonful of salt (9 grams) to a litre of water (0.9% solution of saline). Since this is isotonic with E.C.F. it is known as "Normal saline" - it contains 154 mmols of sodium and 154 mmols of chloride. Ten ml of molar KCl contains 10 mmols of potassium and 10 mmols of chloride.

Four Electrolyte Solutions Used in Surgery

Of the four electrolyte solutions which are used in normal surgical practice there are two which are used to *replace fluid lost* from the body. (e.g. vomiting, diarrhoea, small bowel contents, bile, pancreatic juice) and two solutions which are used to provide *normal daily maintenance requirements.*

Replacement Solutions

Normal Saline plus 10 mls molar KCl. This solution provides 154 mmol sodium, 164 mmol chloride and 10 mmol potassium in 1L of water - this solution is used for the replacement of abnormal losses of gastric fluid.

Plasmalyte. This solution contains 130 mmols of sodium, 103 mmols of chloride, 27 mmols of bicarbonate, 4 mmols of potassium. It is used for replacement of all gastrointestinal losses from the ampulla of Vater down. It is also used to replace volume after extensive dissections, and in burns, sepsis and shock.

Maintenance Solutions

1/5th Normal Saline Plus KCl - This solution contains only 1/5th of the sodium content of "normal saline". It is also called 0.18% saline with dextrose (to make it isotonic) and KCl. One litre of this solution contains 30 mmols sodium, 42 g of dextrose (168 kcal) and 20 mmols of potassium. Two and a half litres of this fluid provide the daily maintenance requirements of water and electrolyte for a 70 Kg patient.

1/5 th Normal Saline Without KCl - Potassium should not be given to postoperative patients and those with renal failure. Two litres of this fluid which is the same as the above solution but without potassium provides the maintenance requirements for a 70 Kg man on the first postoperative day.

Prescribing Fluid and Electrolytes for Surgical Patients

These prescriptions are for a 70 Kg normal adult and should be adjusted according to body weight and obesity.

Maintenance
2.5 litres of 1/5 th normal saline plus KCl

The First Day Post Operation
2 litres 1/5th Normal Saline without KCl.

Abnormal Losses
-Normal Saline + 10 mls molar KCl for gastric losses
-Plasmalyte for all other losses from the gastrointestinal tract or interstitial fluid,
Each litre of abnormal loss is replaced with a litre of the appropriate solution.

Replacement of Pre Existing Deficits
The patient is examined carefully and the deficit is categorise as being *mild*, *moderate* or *severe* according to table 4. The fluid "deficit" is then taken from this table and adjustments are made according to the patient's weight and degree of obesity. Remember "the more fat the less lean" or the fatter the patient the lesser will be his/her fluid and electrolyte requirements. Replacement is with an extracellular fluid substitute: 'Normal Saline' if the deficit is due to gastric lossess. Plasmalyte for all other deficits.

Special Note
No potassium should be given if the patient is in renal failure or the urine output is less than 20 mls/hour.

NUTRITION

Common to all surgical disease are three metabolic processes. There is metabolism of fat for energy, catabolism of protein to provide glucose for tissues that cannot use fat as an energy source (e.g. brain ; healing tissues) and there is an expansion of extra cellular water.Thus the patient with chronic surgical disease presents with deficits in body stores of fat and protein - i.e. he/she suffers to some degree from protein energy malnutrition. If sepsis is present as well stores of body protein may be profoundly depleted. It is important to understand that patients suffer few ill effects from depleted fat stores but losses of protein always impact on physiological function. For example severe protein depletion has been shown to impair respiratory function, skeletal muscle function, wound healing and immune function. It is for this reason that malnourished surgical patients awaiting or recovering from major surgery who have clinical evidence of impending or actual physiological impairments are treated by enteral or parenteral nutrition.

Nutritional Requirements

Surgical patients require more energy and protein than normal subjects. Most non septic patients will gain protein if 40 kcals/kg/day and 0.3 g N/kg/day are administered.

It should be noted though that it is almost impossible for septic patients to gain protein. These requirements are the same whether the nutrients are administered enterally or by the intravenous route.

Enteral Nutrition

Malnourished patients with a functioning small intestine are treated by the continuous instillation of a liquid defined formula diet. A fine nasogastric or jejunal tube is inserted and a commercially available balanced liquid diet is continuously pumped into the intestine.

Parenteral Nutrition

When the gastrointestinal tract is *blocked, fistulated, severely inflamed, too short or simply cannot cope* then nutritional therapy is provided by the intravenous route. Solutions comprising synthetic amino acids, dextrose, fat, appropriate electrolytes, trace elements and vitamins are mixed in the hospital pharmacy and supplied to the ward in large transparent 3L bags. The nutrient solution is infused via a volumetric infusion pump through a subclavian catheter into the superior vena cava. This is a complex procedure requiring skilled medical and nursing staff who adhere to a very strict protocol to prevent complications. The most important complication is infection of the central venous catheter which may be fatal if unrecognized.

SHOCK AND ITS THERAPY

Shock is the state in which vital tissues are inadequately perfused and the common feature is a reduction in the effective circulating blood volume with resulting impairment of ventricular filling and cardiac output. There are a number of different types of which three are the most important - *hypovolaemic shock, cardiogenic shock and septic shock.*

Recognition of Shock

In the early stages of shock, urine output drops, the patient becomes drowsy or confused (reflecting decreased perfusion of the brain), while the blood pressure remains normal. Other signs are a cool skin, a weak fast pulse and tachypnoea. It is only in the latter stages that the blood pressure falls. Adequate treatment in the early stages will prevent the progress of early shock to the frank shock state.

Hypovolaemic Shock

The key to management of hypovolaemic shock is volume *replacement* and control of *bleeding* by direct pressure, surgery or various interventional radiological or endoscopic procedures.

"Normal Saline" or Plasmalyte (*crystalloids*) are initially used for replacement. *Colloid* solutions are then given such as Haemaccel(a 3% solution of gelatin in physiological saline) and SPPS. As soon as blood is ready it is used in generous measure. With massive transfusions clotting factors must also be given.

A urinary catheter and central line are also inserted so as to monitor progress of fluid replacement and response of the patient to resuscitation.

Definitive management depends upon the lesion causing the bleeding but often it involves surgical intervention.

Cardiogenic Shock (Myocardial Infarction)

The diagnosis is usually apparent from the history and examination. Management is basic life support and management of arrhythmias as they occur. Thrombolytic agents now have an important role in myocardial infarction.

Septic Shock

This may occur in any infection and is thought to be due to the release of foreign polysaccharides or proteins. It is usually due to gram negative endotoxins from E.coli, Klebsiella, Proteus and Psuedomonas. It may occur with or without signs of infection such as chills, rigors, and pyrexia. Patients may present with so-called 'hot shock' with increased cardiac output and reduced vascular resistance. However, as the condition progresses cardiac output falls with a rising peripheral resistance (cold shock). Septic shock leads quickly to organ failure and carries a high mortality. Treatment is by volume resuscitation, broad spectrum antibiotics,and surgical drainage of sepsis. If organ failure develops the patient is admitted to the Department of Critical Care for respiratory support,cardiovascular support, the administration of inotropes and treatment of renal failure.

Other Forms of Shock

It is important to differentiate shock due to causes other than those above. In this context it is helpful to observe the neck veins. The above conditions (except cardiogenic shock) are all characterised by empty neck veins. Full neck veins imply an intrathoracic lesion, such as tension pneumothorax or cardiac tamponade. These must be dealt with as soon as they are recognized. *It also must be remembered that an important cause of shock on surgical wards is pulmonary embolism.*

FURTHER READING FOR INTEREST

Cushieri, A; Giles, G.R.; Moosa A.R.: Essential Surgical Practice. 2nd Edition, 1988. Wright, London. Pp 109-131

FURTHER READING FOR FINALS

Way,L.W.: Current Surgical Diagnosis and Treatment. 8th Edition, 1988. Appleton and Lange. Pp 174-176, 181-186

NOTES

Tutorial 4

The Acute Abdomen

Many patients who have had severe abdominal pain for greater than 6 hours will have a condition of surgical importance. If the condition is severe enough to warrant admission to hospital then the patient is said to have an *acute abdomen*.

INVESTIGATION OF THE PATIENT WITH THE ACUTE ABDOMEN

Diagnostic research has shown that more than seventy percent of patients who present with the acute abdomen can have an accurate diagnosis made if a good clinical history is taken and a proper physical examination is performed. The following schema is recommended:

History of Pain
   Obtain a clear history of the patient's pain by asking the patient these key questions:

1. What were you doing when the pain came on?
2. Where was the pain when it started?
3. Has the pain shifted?(remember peritoneo -cutaneous pain)
4. Have you had this pain before?

Obtain a full description of the pain (Ryles 10 questions)

1. Character
2. Severity
3. Situation
4. Localisation
5. Radiation
6. Duration
7. Frequency
8. Times of occurrence
9. Aggravating factors
10. Relieving factors

Ask about vomiting.

Ask about bowel habit and the passage of flatus (in complete bowel obstruction the patient does not pass flatus).

Ask about urinary or menstrual symptoms.

Remember 'Colic' - Colic occurs when there is an abnormal distention of a hollow organ and the pain has the following three characteristics:
- very severe
- makes patient restless
- makes the patient vomit

Having ascertained these features one should be able to lucidly describe the characteristics of the patient's abdominal pain.

Physical Examination

Examine the patient thoroughly. The following points are very important:

> *Inspection* - Watch the patient as he/she lies in bed, is he/she febrile, or hyper-metabolic? Is he /she lying still or is he/she restless? Look at the abdomen to see if it moves with respiration (in peritonitis the abdomen looks rigid). If the abdomen is distended look to see if this is localised (eg gallbladder or appendix mass), or generalised as in small bowel obstruction (central) or large bowel obstruction (in the flanks).

> *Palpation* - with a warm hand, very lightly at first, feel for areas of tenderness. The sine qua non of peritonitis is *rebound tenderness*. Then, deep tenderness is felt for - exquisite deep tenderness over *McBurney's point* is usually due to appendicitis.

> *Percussion* - for free air (as in perforation) or intralumenal air as in intestinal obstruction.

> *Auscultation* - the character of the bowel sounds is noted: high pitched bowel sounds indicate mechanical obstruction of the intestine; absent bowel sounds indicate peritonitis.

SOME IMPORTANT CAUSES OF THE ACUTE ABDOMEN

Acute Appendicitis

<u>History</u>
The patient is usually a young adult, but may be of any age. Usually there is a history

of central abdominal pain which has moved to the right iliac fossa over a period of hours. The patient is usually nauseated and may find it difficult to walk properly because of abdominal tenderness.

Examination
The patient has a modest fever and usually the tongue is coated. Inspection of the abdomen may show some rigidity over the right side. The patient almost always is exquisitely tender over McBurney's point or on rectal examination (Pelvic Appendicitis).

Diagnosis
This is essentially clinical but ultrasound is being used increasingly to diagnose appendicitis to distinguish it from inflammations of the ileo-caecal area (Yersinia).

Treatment
In order to understand the treatment of appendicitis it is helpful to recall the pathophysiology of the condition. For the first 24 hours the appendix is inflamed, distended and tense. After this time, over the next 2-3 days, the inflamed appendix becomes surrounded by omentum. This is known as an appendix mass.

Next, the appendix ruptures and forms an abscess within the surrounding omentum (appendix abscess). In the very old and the very young, omentum may not surround the appendix and generalised peritonitis is a possibility.

Appendicectomy must be performed in the early phases. If an appendix mass is discovered it is treated by nasogastric aspiration, antibiotics and intravenous fluids followed by removal of the appendix some months later. An appendix abscess, when shown to be present by ultrasound, is treated by percutaneous drainage. Some months later the appendix is removed.

Acute Cholecystitis

History
The patient is often a middle aged woman who has had previous attacks of biliary colic, or right upper quadrant pain which have resolved spontaneously. On this occasion, however, the pain has remained fixed in the right upper quadrant and extreme tenderness has developed. She has become generally unwell with fever.

Examination
The patient is toxic and prefers to lie still. The right upper abdomen does not move with respiration. There is tenderness and rebound and possibly a mass in the right

upper quadrant. Murphy's sign (see Tutorial 5) can usually be elicited.

Diagnosis
Ultrasound shows stones in a distended thick walled gallbladder.

Treatment
The treatment is antibiotics, nasogastric aspiration and surgery on the first available elective operating list. Occasionally the gallbladder perforates and the patient suffers from the very serious condition of *biliary peritonitis* which requires urgent surgery.

Perforated Duodenal Ulcer

Perforated duodenal ulcers are much more common than perforated gastric ulcers.

History
About two thirds of patients have a history suggestive of a chronic duodenal ulcer. The patient presents with a sudden, catastrophic upper abdominal pain.

Examination
The patient is unable to move and has a rigid abdomen. Occasionally it will be possible to detect absence of the normal area of liver dullness due to the presence of free air in the peritoneal cavity. Pelvic tenderness may be elicited on rectal examination.

N.B. - Beware the *period of illusion* which occurs 3-6 hours after the perforation. Rigidity and rebound tenderness may lessen because the outpouring of peritoneal fluid in response to the inflammation diminishes the degree of peritoneal irritation.

Diagnosis
The diagnosis is confirmed by the presence of free air under the diaphragm seen on an erect chest film or lateral decubitus film and, in difficult cases, by the use of a gastrograffin swallow.

Treatment
Treatment is by the passage of a nasogastric tube, intravenous antibiotics, resuscitation with normal saline, and urgent surgery. Surgery consists of peritoneal toilet, patching the perforation with omentum and a parietal cell vagotomy, when the ulcer is chronic.

Acute Pancreatitis

Acute Pancreatitis is usually caused by one of two conditions - gallstones or alcohol. Other causes are rare.

History
The patient presents with severe epigastric pain passing through to the back, often associated with profuse vomiting.

Examination
The patient is very unwell and has epigastric tenderness. In severe cases, the patient may be hypovolaemic and in respiratory distress.

Diagnosis
The diagnosis is confirmed by measurement of the serum amylase which is normally above 1000 IU (Amylase levels are often raised in acute gangrenous cholecystitis, bowel obstruction and perforated ulcer, but it is rare to have values above 1000 IU). As pancreatitis can be caused by gallstones a search for these is made with ultrasound. A C.T. scan may be done to assess the degree of pancreatic inflammation.

Treatment
This is best understood by considering the pathophysiology of the condition. Most patients who present with acute pancreatitis have a diffuse *oedematous swelling* of the pancreas. This usually resolves spontaneously within 8 days. More serious cases have *partial necrosis* within the pancreas and the course is more severe and more prolonged. Rarely, the whole pancreas undergoes *haemorrhagic necrosis*: in this situation vasoactive peptides are released and *multiorgan failure* may result. Haemorrhagic necrosis has a high mortality.

Treatment is always conservative at first and for oedematous or mild pancreatitis it is supportive with intravenous fluids(Plasmalyte), naso-gastric suction and pain relief. If there is a prolonged and more severe clinical course, and gallstones have been demonstrated, endoscopic sphincterotomy is performed. In haemorrhagic pancreatitis surgery may be performed to debride the necrotic pancreas.

Complications of Acute Pancreatitis
Pseudocyst or Abscess - Occasionally acute pancreatitis will result in the formation of a *pseudocyst* in the lesser sac. Necrotic pancreas may develop into an abscess. Ultrasound guided percutaneous drainage is used to treat both of these conditions.

Small Bowel Obstruction

Small bowel obstruction is most often caused by *adhesions* which have developed after a previous operation. Obstruction of a loop of small bowel in the neck of a hernial sac is another common cause. All other causes are uncommon.

History
The patient presents with periumbilical small bowel (green apple) colic. He/she rolls around the bed when a spasm comes on but lies still and relaxes when the spasm subsides and disappears.

Examination
The patient is vomiting, not passing flatus and has central abdominal distension. Bowel sounds are active and high pitched and the abdomen is resonant to percussion. Rebound tenderness suggests that the small bowel is strangulated. It is important to search for abdominal scars, hernias and abdominal masses.

Diagnosis
The surgeon asks three questions:
Is there an obstruction?
An erect or lateral decubitus plain x-ray film is taken of the abdomen to answer this question. These films will show fluid levels when the bowel is distended (the only other conditions in which fluid levels are seen are in babies, gastroenteritis and in patients who have had a recent enema).

If so, where is the obstruction?
A supine abdominal film may show the level of the obstruction by the air outline of the distended intestine. Remember the ileum is 'featureless'.

Is the small bowel strangulated?
If there is tenderness on abdominal palpation or rebound tenderness, strangulation is suspected. A rising pulse may indicate strangulation.

Treatment
Initial management is placement of a nasogastric tube to decompress the stomach, fluid and electrolyte replacement and pain relief. If strangulation of the small bowel cannot be exluded (and very often it cannot) then an operation to find the cause and relieve the obstruction is required.

Large Bowel Obstuction

There are three usual causes of large bowel obstruction. By far the most common is obstruction of the left colon by an adenocarcinoma. A stricture secondary to chronic diverticular inflammation or a volvulus are rarer causes of large bowel obstruction.

History
The patient presents with hypogastric green apple colic and obstipation.

Examination
The abdomen is distended particularly in the flanks. The bowel sounds are active and high pitched.

Diagnosis
As with small bowel obstruction diagnosis is aided by plain abdominal X ray films. A rectal examination and sigmoidoscopy are performed to see if there is a distal carcinoma but more often an urgent barium enema makes the diagnosis.

Treatment
Treatment is directed at relieving the distention and removing the obstructing lesion. In left sided colonic cancer the bowel containing the cancer is removed and a proximal colostomy is performed. Some weeks later colonic continuity is restored. This operation was first devised by Professor Henri Hartmann (1860-1952) of Paris. Nowadays any operation on the recto-sigmoid in which the lesion is removed, the rectal stump oversewn and a proximal left iliac fossa colostomy is constructed is called a 'Hartmann's Procedure'. Volvulus may be untwisted and decompressed with a colonoscope.

Acute Diverticulitis

Diverticular disease is common in the sigmoid colon and is usually asymtomatic. It may, however, become complicated and present as an acute abdomen:

Diverticulitis
In this condition the diverticulae have become inflamed. This produces symptoms and signs similar to acute appendicitis but in the left lower quadrant of the abdomen.

Pericolic Abscess
The diverticulae may perforate locally - a single diverticulum may perforate and become surrounded with omentum - this results in a pericolic abscess which may be

drained percutaneously under ultrasound guidance.

Free Perforation
Perforation into the peritoneal cavity may cause *faecal peritonitis*, a condition which has a high mortality. Treatment is surgical and consists of peritoneal toilet and Hartmann's Procedure, i.e. removal of that part of the sigmoid colon which contains the perforated diverticulum and formation of a colostomy. The distal end of the colon is oversewn. Some months later the two ends are anastomosed together and intestinal continuity is restored.

Other Causes of the Acute Abdomen

Renal Colic
This is caused by a stone passing through the ureter. The patient is seized with excruciating loin pain, often radiating into the scrotum. The pain is constant with knife like exacerbations and he/she is unable to lie still and writhes in bed. In ninety percent of cases a stone can be seen on plain x-ray lying along the line of the ureter. Most ureteric stones pass spontaneously.

Ruptured Abdominal Aortic Aneurysm (AAA)
In a patient with a pulsatile epigastric or umbilical mass and abdominal pain the diagnosis is ruptured or bleeding AAA until proven otherwise. The pain is severe, constant, in the centre of the abdomen and radiates through to the back. On examination a tender expansive pulsation can be felt. The patient has the general signs of massive blood loss - pallor, sweating, stertorious bleeding, tachycardia and hypotension. Treatment is immediate laparotomy and replacement of the diseased aorta with a graft.

Acute Ischaemia
Mesenteric ischaemia produces severe abdominal pain, out of all proportion to the physical findings. This condition has a bad prognosis.

Ectopic Pregnancy
This must be suspected in every woman of childbearing age with abdominal pain. The diagnosis is suggested by a period of amenorrhoea, colicky abdominal pain and vaginal bleeding. Bimanual examination may reveal a uterus smaller than would be expected for dates and a tender mass in one or the other fornix. Referred shoulder tip pain results from irritation of the diaphragm by intraperitoneal blood. A ruptured ectopic pregnancy can be a catastrophic event with the patient presenting in shock. *It is a surgical emergency and immediate transfusion and operation are imperative.*

FURTHER READING FOR INTEREST

Silen,W.: Cope's Early Diagnosis of Acute Abdomen. 15th Edition. Oxford University Press, 1979.

FURTHER READING FOR FINALS

Way,L.W.: Current Surgical Diagnosis and Treatment. 8th Edition. 1988 Appleton and Lange , pp 393-403, 556-560, 498-502,446-448, 522-529, 568-572,592-594, 606-611, 849-853, 580-582, 898-899.

NOTES

Tutorial 5

Surgical (Obstructive) Jaundice

Jaundice is a syndrome characterized by hyperbilirubinaemia and deposition of bile pigments in the skin and mucous membranes resulting in a yellow appearance of the patient. You will see it commonly on surgical wards. In this tutorial we discuss the surgical aspects of jaundice, but not the wide range of infectious, haematological and other medical causes of jaundice.

CLASSIFICATION

It is helpful to divide jaundice into *surgical* (post-hepatic) jaundice and *medical* (prehepatic and hepatic) jaundice.

Surgical Jaundice

Post hepatic (obstructive, cholestatic) jaundice is usually called *surgical jaundice* which is important to recognize because it is usually correctable. The underlying cause is an obstruction of the biliary tree, as a result of which bilirubin is unable to enter the GI tract and the *stools become pale*. The *urine is dark* or tea coloured because it contains bilirubin in the water soluble conjugated form. Bile salts in the skin cause *severe itch* - one of the hallmarks of surgical jaundice.

Medical Jaundice

There are two types:

Prehepatic Jaundice

The hyperbilirubinaemia usually comes from haemolysis or breakdown of large haematomas. The bilirubin, not yet conjugated in the liver, is insoluble and therefore it does not appear in the urine (*acholuric jaundice*).

Hepatic

The cause of the hyperbilirubinaemia is hepatocellular damage due to infectious hepatitis, alcoholic liver disease, primary biliary cirrhosis, sepsis, or metabolic abnormalities.

PATHOLOGY OF SURGICAL JAUNDICE

There are three causes of obstruction of the biliary tree:

Stones

By far the most common.

Tumours

Nearly always malignant and usually associated with a poor prognisis. The commonest tumour causing obstruction is *adenocarcinoma of the head of the pancreas*. Occasionally tumours occur in the bile ducts themselves.

Strictures

Rare causes of surgical jaundice. Most are secondary to operative trauma to the duct. Occasionally they are due to sclerosing cholangitis - a progressive disease which causes multiple strictures throughout the biliary tract. In 75% of cases this disease is associated with ulcerative colitis.

PATHOGENESIS OF GALLSTONES

Cholesterol Stones

These account for about 75% of gallstones. Cholesterol, lecithin and bile salts exist in a super saturated solution in the gallbladder even in many normal subjects. If there is a relative deficiency in bile salts, cholesterol or lecithin, crystals may precipitate, aggregate and form stones. This is, of course, a vast over simplification and a number of other factors are now beginning to emerge as important in the development of cholesterol stones. These include a reduction in phospholipid vesicles, the presence of aggregating and antiaggregating substances and the presence of biliary sludge which may act as a nidus for infection. Ultrasound shows sludge in the gallbladder during starvation and pregnancy.

Pigment Stones

In New Zealand, pigment stones account for about 25% of gallstones and they are predisposed to by haemolysis, bile stasis and cirrhosis. Approximately half are radioopaque due to their calcium content. They are composed of a dense mixture of bacteria and their breakdown products and large amounts of bilirubin and bile acids.

CLINICAL PRESENTATIONS OF SURGICAL JAUNDICE

Gallstones

Jaundice *presenting with pain* is usually caused by gallstones. In New Zealand 12% of women between 40 and 50 years of age have gallstones and 25% of women over the age of 60 years have gallstones.The prevalence is less in men. As the number of patients requiring cholecystectomy is less common than this it is clear that many patients with gallstones are never troubled by them.

Biliary Colic and Cholecystitis

When a gallstone becomes impacted in the neck of the gallbladder or in the cystic duct, distension occurs and the patient is seized with a *severe unremitting pain (Biliary Colic)*, which causes her to *roll around*. The pain is so severe that it is usually associated with *vomiting*.

If the obstruction is not relieved, the gallbladder becomes inflamed by the chemical action of bile salts. Later, infection supervenes (usually E.coli), the gallbladder wall becomes reddened, thickened and oedematous, and the patient is said to have *acute cholecystitis*. Examination reveals that the patient is tender in the right upper quadrant when asked to breathe in. This sign was first described by Dr John B Murphy (1857-1916), the famous Chicago Professor of Surgery who was trained in Vienna under Billroth. The sign is the result of the tense and inflamed gallbladder being brought down to touch the fingers on inspiration. Patients with acute cholecystitis have a fever and a leucocytosis and often have mild jaundice (bilirubin never greater than three times normal). Ultrasound shows stones in the gallbladder associated with a thickened and oedematous wall.Although acute cholecystitis usually settles with conservative treatment, on occasion the gall bladder may perforate, either locally into the duodenum or generally into the peritoneal cavity causing biliary peritonitis, a condition with a high mortality.

Other Clinical Manifestations of Gallstones

Stones originating in the gall bladder may also pass into and impact in the common bile duct giving rise to surgical jaundice. Stones in the duct usually become infected, causing inflammation of the biliary tree (cholangitis) .The three cardinal signs of Cholangitis are *pain, jaundice, and chills with fever* (Charcot's Triad). These signs were first described by Dr Jean Charcot (1825-1893) of Paris who created a great neurological clinic. His lectures on neuropathic joints and the cardinal signs of cholangitis associated with a gallstone impacted in the common bile duct were attended by immense audiences. He also pointed out the serious implications of untreated cholangitis which may cause septicaemia and death,

Not infrequently, small stones from the gallbladder may migrate into the common bile duct and cause pancreatitis by blocking the ampulla of Vater, allowing biliary lecithin into the pancreatic duct under pressure. Phospholipase A acting on biliary lecithin forms lysolecithin which when mixed with bile salts is known to cause severe pancreatitis,

Tumours

Tumours of the head of the pancreas or within the common or hepatic bile ducts present with *painless jaundice*. This is an intense cholestatic jaundice with pale stools, dark urine and intense itch. Often the itch comes on before the jaundice. One important sign in differentiating a tumour from stones was described by Dr Ludwig Courvoisier (1843-1918), a famous Basle surgeon who founded the specialty of hepato-biliary surgery. His law (Courvoisier's Law) states that when the common bile duct is obstructed by a stone, dilatation of the gallbladder is rare. When the duct is obstructed in some other way, dilatation is common. The reason for this is that if the obstruction is due to gallstones then the gallbladder which produces those gallstones will have been subjected to chronic inflammation amd hence is fibrotic and inelastic. It is therefore unable to dilate if obstruction of the duct supervenes.

Strictures

Strictures usually present with Charcot's Triad. Because most strictures are the result of surgical misadventure surgeons take exceptional care to dissect out the junction of the cystic duct and common bile duct when performing cholecystectomy. If damage occurs to the bile duct and a stricture develops as a consequence the patient may be troubled by bouts of cholangitis for the rest of his /her life.

INVESTIGATIONS

Liver Function Tests

The term *liver function test* refers to a serologic test that evaluates an aspect of liver function. Such tests are best interpreted within the setting of the total clinical picture. In surgical jaundice, besides a raised conjugated bilirubin in the blood, *serum alkaline phosphatase* is raised and *coagulation factors* are low.

Alkaline Phosphatase

May originate from the ducts of the liver and levels rise when these are blocked. Hence marked elevations are seen in patients with surgical jaundice.

Coagulation Factors

With obstruction of the biliary tree bile salts fail to enter the small intestine, critical micellar concentrations are not reached and dietary fat is not absorbed. As a result, fat soluble vitamin K, essential for normal coagulation, is also not absorbed and coagulation becomes deranged. It is for this reason that patients with surgical jaundice are given intramuscular vitamin K to restore coagulation to normal before an operative procedure is embarked upon.

Serum Transaminases

Are used as indicators of hepatocellular damage. Aspartate amino transferase (AST) and alanine amino transferase (ALT) are the transaminases commonly measured.
ALT is found primarily in the liver but AST is present in many tissues as well including the heart, kidney, skeletal muscle and brain. Striking elevations of these transaminases are seen when the hepatocytes have been damaged, such as occurs in hepatitis and hepatocellular failure. In patients with extra hepatic obstruction, transaminase levels are usually low.

Imaging the Biliary Tree

Plain X rays

These are not very helpful. Only 10% of gallstones are radio opaque.

Cholecystogram

Oral contrast is taken in the evening and abdominal X rays are taken the next morning. If the gall bladder is functioning normally and contains stones these are outlined by the contrast. If contrast has not entered the gall bladder on two separate occasions (called non opacification) then the gall bladder is said to be non functioning and there is a 95% chance that gallstones are present.

Ultrasound

This is a very accurate and non invasive way of imaging the gallbladder when gallstones are suspected. It is also helpful in diagnosing acute cholecystitis. It is not so good for imaging tumours or stones in the common bile duct particularly at its lower end.

H.I.D.A. scan

Technetium labelled iminodiacetic acid (I.D.A.) derivatives are injected, taken up by the liver and concentrated in the bile. If the gallbladder does not fill there is a 95% chance that the cystic duct is blocked.

Computerised Tomography (CT)

An expensive way of looking at the biliary tree. It can be very helpful for identifying and characterising tumours, particularly those in the head of the pancreas.

Endoscopic Retrograde Cholangiopancreatography (ERCP)

The ampulla of Vater is cannulated via a fibreoptic endoscope and dye is injected into the biliary tree and pancreatic ducts. This is the best way of outlining the biliary tree and is helpful for identifying stones, tumours and strictures.

Percutaneous Transhepatic Cholangiography (PTC)

A fine needle is introduced percutaneously through the liver into a dilated bile duct and contrast is injected to fill the biliary tree. This technique is useful for looking at the proximal biliary tree and demonstrates obstruction well, particularly when it is above the common hepatic duct.

Intraoperative Cholangiography

This is routinely performed during cholecystectomy to check that there are no common duct stones. The contrast is introduced by the surgeon into the biliary tree through the cystic duct stump.

Choledochoscopy

The common bile duct can be visualised during operation by the surgeon by using a very fine endoscope. This is routinely done after operative exploration of the common bile duct to ensure that all stones have been removed.

T Tube Cholangiography

Whenever the surgeon has explored the common bile duct, a T Tube is left in the choledochotomy incision to prevent leakage of bile. On the 8th postoperative day dye is passed down the T Tube to ensure that no stones have been left behind. If all is clear, the tube is removed.

TREATMENT

Stones

There are four ways of managing these:

Surgery

For stones in the gallbladder which are causing symptoms (ie biliary colic or cholecystitis) the best management is removal of the gallbladder (cholecystectomy). In patients with acute cholecystitis cholecystectomy is best done within a few days of onset.

Chemical

There have been many attempts to dissolve cholesterol gallstones medically. Bile salts are taken orally for 6 months to 2 years. Although small stones may dissolve, they usually recur when the treatment is stopped.

Endoscopic Sphincterotomy

When a stone is present in the common bile duct (jaundice or cholangitis) it may be removed by transecting the ampullary sphincter via an endoscope. The source of the stone, the gall bladder, is usually removed by surgery at a later date but in elderly patients cholecystectomy is not usually necessary.

Lithotripsy

A possible new treatment for some gallstones, at present under evaluation. The patient, without an anaesthetic, is bombarded with high energy sound waves which are beamed on to the stone, which disintegrates.

Tumours

These are resected if possible, although most malignant tumours of the head of the pancreas are incurable at the time of presentation. In these circumstances the surgeon has the choice of bypassing the obstruction (choleycystojejunostomy) or passing a silastic stent through the obstruction via an endoscope. Tumours at the ampulla or in the bile duct, if small, are best resected using the procedure described in 1935 by Dr Allan Whipple of New York. He discovered that it was possible to reverse the bleeding tendency in jaundiced patients by first performing the fairly minor procedure of cholecystogastrostomy. Because vitamin K could then be absorbed again, clotting returned to normal, enabling the major procedure of pancreaticoduodenectomy(Whipple's Procedure) to be performed without fear of torrential bleeding.

Strictures

These are either dealt with by surgery (which can be very difficult) or by the endoscopic placement of a silastic stent.

FURTHER READING FOR INTEREST

Chopra,S, Griffin,P.H. (1988): Laboratory Tests and Diagnostic Proceedures in Evaluation of Liver Disease. Am J Med 79, 221

Norrby, S. et al. (1983): Early or Delayed Cholecystectomy in Acute Cholecystitis? A Clinical Trial. Br J Surg 70, 163

FURTHER READING FOR FINALS

Way. L.W.: Current Surgical Diagnosis and Treatment. 8th Edition, 1988 Appleton and Lange. Pp 492-507, 534-537.

NOTES

Tutorial 6

Haematemesis, Melaena and Peptic Ulcer Disease

DEFINITIONS

Haematemesis is the vomiting of blood. Its source is usually proximal to the ligament of Trietz (D J Flexure) and usually indicates a rapidly bleeding lesion. Vomiting of old blood which has been in the stomach for some time resembles *coffee grounds*. *Melaena* is the passage of pitch black stools. The colour and characteristic smell are due to bacterial degradation of blood which originates in the stomach, duodenum or small bowel.

AETIOLOGY OF HAEMATEMESIS AND MELAENA

Peptic Ulcer Disease	
Duodenal Ulcer	30%
Gastric Ulcer	25%
Gastric Erosion	20%
Mallory Weiss Tear	10%
Oesophageal Varices	10%
Gastric Cancer	5%
and other uncommon causes	

PEPTIC ULCER DISEASE

Peptic Ulcer Disease is the end result of acid-pepsin action on vulnerable gastric or duodenal epithelium. The most common sites for ulcers are the *first part of the duodenum* and the *lesser curve of the stomach*.

Pain is the most common presentation. It is usually in the epigastrium and is burning or aching in nature. Some patients complain of a deep hunger sensation. Generally features of the pain do not accurately differentiate between a gastric ulcer and a duodenal ulcer but the pain is often related in some way to food. Ulcers may bleed and present with haematemesis or melaena or the ulcer may cause anaemia without these manifestations. An ulcer may *perforate* through the wall of the stomach or duodenum into the abdominal cavity or posteriorly into the pancreas. Scarring and swelling around a chronic ulcer may cause *obstruction,* just beyond the pylorus.

Pathophysiology

Duodenal Ulcers

These are usually chronic and are associated with high acid secretion and a defect in the duodenal mucus barrier. Recently attention has been focussed upon the presence of Helicobacter pylori, which may reside in metaplastic gastric epithelium near or within a chronic duodenal ulcer and be responsible for ulcer relapse unless the organism is eliminated.

Gastric Ulcers

There are three distinct types of Gastric ulcer:

Type 1
These are associated with low acid production and are found on the lesser curvature, usually near the angular notch just distal to the junction between the parietal cell mass and the antral mucosa. These ulcers are probably the result of a weakened mucosa secondary to regurgitation of duodenal juice.

Type 2
These are found in association with duodenal ulcers and are also found on the lesser curve of the stomach. The initiating factor is the duodenal ulcer causing some degree of antral distension - a potent stimulus for gastrin release.

Type 3
These are found in the antrum and are most often secondary to the use of non steroidal anti inflammatory medications.

Antral gastritis is a separate entity and may be caused by H.pylori.

Gastric Cancer

Important points about cancer - while duodenal carcinoma is very rare, gastric carcinoma is not. For this reason *all gastric ulcers must be biopsied to ensure malignancy is not present.* Gastric carcinoma may present in exactly the same way as a benign gastric ulcer and look similar to it. If a gastric ulcer presents on the greater curve of the stomach it is likely to be an adenocarcinoma.

Diagnosis

History and physical examination, although helpful, have a low rate of sensitivity and specificity. For this reason, other diagnostic procedures are required for patients who present with symptoms suggestive of peptic ulcer disease or with haematemesis or melaena. There are two imaging procedures that are commonly used to make the diagnosis:

Barium Meal

This outlines the ulcer crater and deformities produced by ulcers of the stomach or duodenum. The sensitivity and specificity is high. Barium studies are of special use when bleeding is not the presenting problem.

Endoscopy

This is the most commonly used diagnostic tool for peptic ulcer disease. It is of particular value in determining the source of gastroduodenal bleeding.

Treatment

Peptic Ulcer Disease may be divided into 2 groups for the purposes of management:

Uncomplicated Peptic Ulcer Disease

The management of uncomplicated disease is medical and involves the removal of predisposing factors such as smoking, non steroidal anti inflammatory medicines and the amelioration of environmental stress. Medicines used are the H2 antagonists (Ranitidine) and cytoprotective agents such as colloidal bismuth (De-Nol).

Complicated Peptic Ulcer Disease

There are 4 major complications of Peptic Ulcer Disease:

Intractability
This is a term used to describe ulcers that cannot be healed by optimal medical measures. Surgery is therefore indicated although its timing differs according to the type of ulcer. In the case of duodenal ulcer, surgery is not undertaken until after a long period (approximately 2 years) of optimal medical management which has failed to relieve symptoms. The procedure is denervation of the parietal cell mass (parietal cell vagotomy, sometimes called highly selective vagotomy). For benign

gastric ulcers, which are more likely to be resistent to medical therapy than duodenal ulcers, surgery is undertaken earlier (6 months to 1 year). The procedure involves removal of the distal half of the stomach (including the ulcer) and a gastro-duodenal anastomosis (Billroth I gastrectomy). This is named after its founder, Dr Theodore Billroth of Vienna, who performed the first succesful gastrectomy in 1881.

Perforation

Most ulcers which perforate, do so from the anterior aspect of the duodenum and cause sudden onset of severe upper abdominal pain secondary to the outpouring of duodenal contents. When suspected a nasogastric tube is passed to empty the stomach of its contents. The diagnosis is confirmed by a plain abdominal X ray (erect or lateral decubitus) which reveals free air in 85% of patients. Treatment is surgical and consists of patching the perforation with omentum and a parietal cell vagotomy if the ulcer is chronic. Gastric ulcers may perforate too, and because there is a high chance of malignancy (approximately 15%), the treatment is a Billroth I gastrectomy.

Obstruction

The management of gastric outlet obstruction is at first medical. The patient may present with a complex fluid and electrolyte disorder - hypochloraemic, hypokalaemic metabolic alkalosis as a result of prolonged vomiting. Remembering that the pathology is twofold - fibrosis which is irreversible, and swelling which is reversible - the principles of management are nasogastric tube aspiration, restoration of electrolyte and fluid balance (normal saline with 10 mmol of potassium per litre of fluid), gut rest and then a slow introduction of a liquid diet and solid food as tolerated. If the patient does not improve rapidly, surgery is proceeded with. The pylorus and first part of the duodenum are widened (pyloroplasty) and the trunks of the vagus nerves are cut to diminish the secretion of acid from the parietal cell mass.

Bleeding

Bleeding from peptic ulceration, once the diagnosis is confirmed by endoscopy, is usually managed medically by restoration of blood volume, bed rest and Ranitidine. Surgery is required in approximately 20% of patients and is based on the following guidelines: In patients over 60 years of age, surgery is performed if a bleeding vessel is identified at endoscopy, if more than 4 units of blood are needed in the first 12 hours, or if the patient rebleeds whilst in hospital. In patients younger than 60, the indications for surgery are a 'bleeder' at endoscopy, a requirement of greater than 8 units of blood in the first 12 hours or 2 rebleeds whilst in hospital. At surgery, the bleeding vessel is found and transfixed with a suture. If there is a duodenal ulcer, then the treatment is the same as for obstruction (truncal vagotomy and pyloroplasty) or if there is a gastric ulcer this is dealt with by a Billroth I gastrectomy.

TREATMENT OF OTHER CAUSES OF HAEMATEMESIS AND MELAENA

Oesophageal Varices

Raised pressure in the portal venous system (portal hypertension) results in the lower oesophageal plexus becoming dilated and varicosed. Bleeding from the varicosities is not uncommon and can sometimes be massive. Treatment is by the endoscopic injection of the varices with sclerosant and the lowering of portal pressure by medical measures.

Gastric Cancer

This does not usually cause severe gastric bleeding. The patient is much more likely to present with weight loss, anaemia and a palpable epigastric mass. Most carcinomas of the stomach in New Zealand present late and the treatment is palliative, i.e. Billroth II Gastrectomy in which the stomach is reconstructed after partial resection by joining the remaining proximal segment to the jejunum.

Mallory Weiss Syndrome

This is bleeding from a tear in the gastric mucosa near its junction with the oesophagus. It is caused by vigorous vomiting. In gastric erosions and Mallory Weiss tears the bleeding is almost always self limiting

STOMACH OPERATIONS

Glossary of Terms

Vagotomy

There are two types of vagotomy

Highly Selective Vagotomy

Only the nerves to the parietal cell mass are cut and the stomach empties normally because the antrum is still innervated

Truncal Vagotomy

Both vagi are divided as they enter the abdomen, i.e. total abdominal vagotomy. The stomach is denervated and therefore does not empty. A drainage procedure is thus required (pyloroplasty or gastro-jejunostomy)

Gastric Resection

There are two types of Gastric Resection:

Partial Gastrectomy

May be antrum only (antrectomy) or 50% of stomach (hemigastrectomy)

Total Gastrectomy

The whole stomach is removed and replaced with a limb of jejunum

Gastric Reconstruction

There are 2 ways of restoring gastro-intestinal continuity after partial resection of the stomach

Billroth I Reconstruction

When the proximal stomach is anastomosed to the first part of the duodenum

Billroth II Reconstruction

When the proximal stomach is anastomosed to a loop of proximal jejunum

FURTHER READING FOR INTEREST

Hunt, P.S. (1984) : Surgical Management of Bleeding Chronic Peptic Ulcer. A 10 year Prospective Study. Ann Surg 199, 144

Venables, C.W. (1986): Mucus, Pepsin and Peptic Ulcer. Gut 27, 233

FURTHER READING FOR FINALS

Way, L.W.: Current Surgical Diagnosis and Management. 8th Edition,1988 . Appleton and Lange. Pp 427-432, 438-452, 454, 471-486.

NOTES

Tutorial 7

Bleeding from the Anus, Rectum and Colon

BLEEDING FROM THE ANUS

Anatomy of the Anal Canal

The anal canal is 4-5cms in length. It is surrounded by two concentric rings of muscle: an inner ring of involuntary muscle - the internal sphincter, and an outer ring of voluntary muscle - the external sphincter. The dentate line is seen as a wavy line in the mucous membrane of the anal canal exactly halfway up the internal sphincter. Above the dentate line there is columnar epithelium - thus no pain is felt in this region. Below the dentate line there is progressively thickening squamous epithelium - thus pain is felt in this area. The internal haemorrhoidal plexus of veins lies in the submucosal layer above the dentate line. This plexus comprises a circle of veins supported by connective tissue cushions. The external haemorrhoidal plexus of veins lies under the skin surrounding the anal verge.

Physical Examination of the Anal Canal

The external sphincter is under voluntary control, whilst the internal sphincter is under involuntary control. During digital rectal examination, one can feel the groove between the edge of the internal sphincter and overlapping external sphincter just inside the anal canal. After about 4 cms the finger reaches the capacious rectum. Posteriorly, a bar is felt in this region, this is the puborectalis sling. This sling pulls forward at the junction of the anus and rectum and provides a shutter mechanism which is the most important factor in continence.

The anal canal is examined via a proctoscope (anoscope in America). This short tube is passed through the anal canal into the lower rectum. It is then slowly withdrawn as the patient strains down. When the opening of the proctoscope reaches the dentate line, the whole of the internal haemorrhoidal plexus can be visualised just above it.

N.B. It should be remembered though that no examination of the anal canal is complete unless the rectum has been examined as well.

Haemorrhoids (Piles)

Some people in some families are born with a deficiency of the connective tissue cushions in which the internal haemorrhoidal plexus of veins is embedded. This predisposes them to haemorrhoids which are simply varicosities (dilated abnormal veins) of the internal plexus. They are prone to occur particularly if there is associated constipation. If the patient is examined in the lithotomy position via a proctoscope, the varicosities can be seen to be present at the 3 o'clock, 7 o'clock and 11 o'clock positions.

There are three degrees of severity:

<u>First degree</u>

Bleeding occurs from the anus after a bowel motion.

<u>Second degree</u>

The varicosed veins fall out after a bowel motion.

<u>Third degree</u>

The varicosed veins stay out of the anal canal after a bowel motion and may thrombose (fourth degree).

In *first degree* haemorrhoids the hard stool coming down the anal canal crushes the veins and as a consequence bright red blood coats the stool or comes just after the stool is passed. These haemorrhoids are common. Almost everyone will have an episode of first degree haemorrhoids at some time in their lives particularly when constipated. Since the varicosities occur beneath the anal canal epithelium above the dentate line, there is no pain associated with internal haemorrhoids.

Patients with *second degree* haemorrhoids have the feeling that a mass has come out of the anus after passing a bowel movement. This mass reduces spontaneously but is associated with a dragging discomfort. These haemorrhoids do not usually bleed.

Patients with *third degree* haemorrhoids have a mass which comes out of the anus and stays out. They are coated with mucus producing epithelium and perianal soiling occurs which is distressing for the patient. These haemorrhoids cause a dragging feeling, perianal tenderness and debilitating dull pain.

Patients with *fourth degree* haemorrhoids have a large thrombosed mass protruding from the anus. The patient may suffer from excruciating pain.

Treatment

First degree haemorrhoids are treated by injecting a sclerosant into the connective tissue cushions at the top of the anal canal. This sclerosant (5% phenol in almond oil) excites fibrosis, increasing the strength of the cushions. Surgeons in the USA put rubber bands on the haemorrhoids, cutting the varicosities off totally (like the process used for removal of lambs' tails).

Second degree haemorrhoids are also treated by the injection of sclerosant. Some advanced second degree piles are treated surgically.

Third and fourth degree haemorrhoids are treated surgically - the varicosed veins are dissected out, tied off and removed. Haemorrhoidectomy is one of the more painful operations of surgery.

External Haemorrhoids (External Anal Haematoma)

This very painful condition occurs as a result of rupture of the veins of the external haemorrhoidal plexus. It may occur during vigorous activity. After a few days the haematoma undergoes fibrosis, but there remains a skin tag at the site. Sometimes the condition is so painful that the haematoma needs to be drained.

Anal Fissures

Anal fissures and haemorrhoids often occur together. A fissure is a tear in the mucus membrane of the anal canal below the dentate line. It usually arises after a hard faecal mass has been passed. Pain occurs during defaecation and as a consequence the patient is reluctant to pass a bowel motion and a chronic self perpetuating cycle can result.

If the fissure becomes chronic, granulation tissue forms a *sentinel pile* and the internal sphincter goes into severe spasm.

There is a history of severe anal pain occurring both during and for some time after passing a motion. Bright red blood coming after the the stool has been passed is usually noticed. Diagnosis of fissure is made by inspection. The patient will be sitting on the edge of his chair. He will have an aching anus which is extremely difficult to examine (shy anus) and an anaesthetic may therefore be required to make a diagnosis. Fissures must be distinguished from anal fistulas. These arise after a perianal or anal abscess has burst onto the skin surrounding the anus. If the skin opening connects with the anal canal then a fistula is said to be present.

Surgical Treatment of Anal Fissure

A lateral *subcutaneous sphincterotomy* should be considered if the fissure remains refractory after pain relief has been given and efforts have been made to regulate the bowel habit. A knife is passed between the external and internal sphincters and the lower portion of the internal sphincter is divided, thus breaking the spasm so that motions can be passed painlessly. The fissure usually heals promptly within three weeks after this minor procedure.

BLEEDING FROM THE RECTUM

Anatomy of the Rectum

The rectum extends from the ano-rectal junction, about 4 cm from the anal verge, to the rectosignmoid junction at 13-15 cm from the anal verge.

Physical Examination of the Rectum

The lower two thirds of the rectum can be examined by the finger (P.R. Examination). A sigmoidoscope (proctoscope in America) is a rigid metal tube about 30 cms long which contains a light source and a lens system and it is the instrument most commonly used to examine the rectum.

Tumours of the Rectum

Tumours of the rectum may bleed. The blood, usually bright red but sometimes clots, mixes with the stool or coats the stool as it is stored in the rectum. This bleeding may arise from:

Benign Tumours of the Rectum (Polyps)

Polyps are small masses of tissue that project into the lumen of the rectum. Most polyps are asymtomatic but the larger the lesion the more likely it is to cause symptoms. Rectal bleeding is by far the commonest complaint - it is usually intermittent and blood flecks the stool. P.R. examination usually fails to detect any abnormality. The diagnosis is therefore made by sigmoidoscopy at which time the polyps are removed and sent for histology. There are 4 types of polyps: *neoplastic, hamartomatous, inflammatory* and *metaplastic* (see below under Benign Tumours of the Colon). Only the neoplastic polyps have malignant potential. Cancer is found in 45% of neoplastic polyps which are greater than 2 cm in diameter.

Malignant Tumours of the Rectum

Adenocarcinoma is the only malignant tumour of the rectum of importance. There is a high incidence of this disease in New Zealand. Over two thirds of these tumours can be felt with the examining finger at which time a hard craggy mass or ulcer is palpated leaving little doubt as to the likely diagnosis. The clinical diagnosis is confirmed by sigmoidoscopy and biopsy. Because these tumours can so often be felt by the finger surgeons teach that in any case of rectal bleeding 'If you don't put your finger in it you will put your foot in it'. Treatment is by *anterior resection* where the tumour containing rectum is removed and the colon is stapled to the remaining low rectum or anal canal. If the cancer invades the puborectalis muscle, the whole rectum is removed together with the anal canal (*abdomino - perineal resection* of the rectum) In this situation the patient is left with a permanent left iliac fossa *colostomy*. Prognosis depends on the pathological stage of the tumour. In 1958, London Pathologist Dr Cuthbert Dukes published his research on the spread of rectal cancer and its effect on prognosis, based on the study of 2,500 operation specimens. The crude 5 year survival for all patients treated by surgical removal of the primary tumour was 50%. When he related the local spread of the tumour to ultimate survival he was able to describe 3 stages.

Dukes' A - the cancer is confined to the bowel wall - 90% 5 year survival
Dukes' B - through bowel wall, no nodal involvement - 60% 5 year survival
Dukes' C - through bowel wall with nodal involvement - 30% 5 year survival

Inflammation of the Rectum (Proctitis)

This is associated with blood mixed in the stool. The stool is usually loose and frequently contains pus and mucus as well.

Proctitis

Diffuse inflammation of the rectal mucosa. When seen with a sigmoidoscope, the mucosa is inflamed, bleeds easily and may be coated with pus. Ulcers may also be seen. If this inflammation is confined to the rectum the condition is called proctitis. If it extends above the rectum it is known as proctocolitis or sometimes just colitis.

Proctitis may be due to a specific infection, Ulcerative Colitis, or Crohn's Disease. Bright blood is mixed in with the stool and the patient usually presents with bloody diarrhoea (up to twelve motions a day). Episodes of proctitis tend to be intermittent- every few months, lasting about 3-6 weeks. The diagnosis is made by sigmoidoscopy and biopsy after exclusion of specific infections by stool culture. Ulcerative colitis and Crohn's proctitis are treated by steroids administered locally via an enema.

BLEEDING FROM THE COLON

Surgical Anatomy of the Colon

Surgeons talk of the sigmoid colon, left colon, transverse colon and right colon because of their distinct blood supply. For surgical treatment of cancer the tumour bearing colon must be resected together with the draining lymphnodes. Since these lymphnodes follow the main colon arteries these resections are described as sigmoid colectomy, left hemicolectomy, transverse colectomy and right hemicolectomy.

Physical Examination of the Colon

This is done either by a double contrast Barium Enema or by a flexible fibre-optic colonoscope.

Tumours of the Colon

<u>Benign Tumours of the Colon</u>

Polyps can occur in any part of the colon. Like the rectum, neoplastic, hamartomatous, inflammatory and metaplastic polyps can occur. Neoplastic polyps (adenomas) are of three histological types which are variations of one histological process - <u>tubular adenomas tubulovillous adenomas and villous adenomas</u>. The potential for cancerous transformation increases with time and is related to the size of the adenomas. Most adenocarcinomas of the large bowel evolve from adenomas. For this reason, all polyps of the colon are removed. A snare, inserted via a colonoscope, is passed around the base of the polyp which is then cauterized. Although it is not uncommon for patients to have several polyps there is a rare but important condition called *"Familial Polyposis"* in which hundreds of polyps may be seen. Cancer develops before the age of 40 in nearly all untreated patients.

Malignant Tumours of the Colon

Adenocarcinoma - New Zealand has one of the highest incidences of carcinoma of the colon in the world, particularly in women. As for the rectum, colon cancer is classified by Duke's classification, and the prognosis is the same as that for the rectum.

Presentation
Patients with right sided cancer of the colon usually present with occult bleeding and anaemia and a right iliac fossa mass may be palpable. Left sided cancer of the colon usually presents with intermittent diarrhoea and constipation, blood mixed in with the stool, or obstruction of the large bowel.

Diagnosis
This is made by barium enema or by colonoscopy.

Treatment
Right hemicolectomy, transverse colectomy, left hemicolectomy or sigmoid colectomy with immediate anastomosis.

Diverticular Disease

This is a disease of Western Society and usually involves the sigmoid colon. It may cause bright red rectal bleeding which is usually selflimiting. The diverticulae may also become inflamed (diverticulitis) and present as a left sided appendicitis or may perforate causing a local abscess (pericolic abscess) or faecal peritonitis.

Angiodysplasia

Submucosal arterio-venous malformations may occur in elderly patients and present with bright red rectal bleeding. Diagnosis is usually made by colonoscopy. When noted these submucosal vascular abnormalities may be coagulated.

Inflammatory Bowel Disease

Loose stools with blood mucus and pus suggest the patient may be suffering from inflammatory bowel disease. Although there are a number of types of inflammatory bowel disease, the commonest are Ulcerative Colitis and Crohn's Disease.

Ulcerative Colitis

Ulcerative colitis always starts in the rectum and progresses proximally. It is limited to the large intestine and is a disease which is histologically confined to the mucosa. It may predispose to cancer if it involves the whole colon over a period of 10 years or more. Treatment is at first medical(Salazopyrin to prevent attacks and steroids to limit attacks) and if this is unsuccessful then surgery may have to be employed. Surgery involves:
-Removal of the anus, rectum and colon with formation of an ileostomy in the right iliac fossa (Panproctocolectomy with permanent ileostomy).
-Removal of the rectum and colon with formation of a new rectum from the ileum (Ileo-anal anastomosis with J Pouch).

Crohn's Colitis

This disease may occur anywhere in the tubular gut and is patchy in its distribution. There are three broad patterns of Crohn's Disease. Jejuno-ileal disease, which has the worst prognosis, ileo-caecal disease which has the best prognosis and Crohn's Colitis. Although the disease may be confined to and involve the whole colon, occurrence localised in the rectum or the ileo-caecal area is more common. Histologically, it is a transmural disease and when it involves the whole colon it may predispose to cancer but this is not as common as it is in ulcerative colitis. Treatment is at first medical but if the colitis becomes severe then *panproctocolectomy* and *ileostomy* is indicated.

FURTHER READING FOR INTEREST

Goligher, J.C.(1983): Surgery of the Anus, Rectum and Colon. 5th Edition, Balliere Tindall

FURTHER READING FOR FINALS

Way, L.W.: Current Surgical Diagnosis and Treatment. 8th Edition, 1988. Appleton and Lange Pp 594-630, 637-644, 573-576

NOTES

Tutorial 8

Swellings of the Thyroid Gland (Goitre) and other Swellings of the Head and Neck

ANATOMY

Head and neck swellings usually occur within existing anatomical structures. The key to diagnosis is therefore an understanding of the principles of the regional anatomy. This includes:

Anterior Triangle of the Neck

The anterior triangle of the neck, where most swellings of the neck occur, is bounded laterally by the anterior margin of the sternomastoid muscle, superiorly by the inferior border of the mandible and medially by the midline. The anterior triangle contains the median visceral column comprising the pharynx, larynx and trachea and the thyroid and parathyroid glands.

Cervical Lymph Nodes

Lymph nodes occur in the suboccipital region, the posterior triangle, and the supra clavicular region. Much more important though are the deep cervical lymph nodes in association with the carotid sheath. Enlargements of these lymph nodes are the commonest cause of swellings in the neck.

The Thyroid Gland

This bilobed gland is not normally palpable and lies deep to the strap muscles in the neck. The recurrent laryngeal nerves supply the intrinsic muscles of the larynx and are closely applied to the posterior aspects of the thyroid lobes. During thyroidectomy the surgeon displays these nerves so that inadvertant damage is avoided.

The Parathyroid Glands

There are usually 4 glands, each weighs about 30-40 mg. Their close approximation to the posterior aspect of the thyroid lobes also makes them vulnerable to damage during thyroidectomy.

The Parotid Gland

The parotid gland lies in front of and below the lower half of the ear. Swellings in the gland may push the ear lobe upwards. The facial nerve passes through the stylo mastoid foramen into the parotid gland which divides it into a superficial and a deep lobe. Since the bulk of the gland is in the superficial lobe this is where most swellings occur. The operation of superficial parotidectomy removes the superficial lobe and preserves the facial nerve. Malignant tumours of the parotid may invade the facial nerve and cause facial paralysis.

SWELLING OF THE THYROID GLAND (GOITRE)

When examining the thyroid gland the student should try to decide if there is *one lump, many lumps or a diffuse enlargement of the whole gland.* He/she must also assess thyroid function and be able to describe the patient as *Thyrotoxic, Hypothyroid or Euthyroid.*

One Lump is Found

This is called a solitary nodule of the thyroid. Ultrasound examination will ascertain if it is *solid* or *cystic.* A radio-nuclide scan will ascertain if the nodule is functioning (warm or *hot*) or non functioning (*cold*).

<u>Solid Thyroid Nodules</u>

Hot Solid Thyroid Nodule
This is a functioning adenoma of the thyroid. It is one cause of thyrotoxicosis. Hot nodules are almost never malignant. Treatment is local removal of the nodule.

Cold Solid Thyroid Nodule
This has 20% chance of being malignant. Most often such a nodule is a benign, *follicular adenoma.* Less often it is a *differentiated thyroid cancer* of either the *papillary* or *follicular* type. Because differentiated thyroid cancer is difficult to diagnose accurately, the treatment of most cold solid thyroid nodules is surgical. The total thyroid lobe containing the tumour is removed together with the isthmus and most of the other lobe. The reason that most of the other lobe is removed is that these tumours are often multicentric. If definitive histology shows the differentiated thyroid cancer to be of the papillary type no further treatment is required except that the patient should continue taking thyroxine for life. This suppresses thyroid stimulating hormone. If the tumour is of the follicular type and seen to be invading blood vessels then the remaining lobe is ablated by radioactive iodine. This renders the

patient hypothyroid at which time a radionuclide scan will show if any thyroid tissue remains. If there is, further radioactive iodine ablation is carried out. A nodule less than 2 cms in diameter which presents in a young person and contains well differentiated thyroid cancer of either type has a benign course.

Many Lumps are Found (Multinodular Goitre)

Multinodular Goitre occurs in patients from iodine poor regions or as a result of prolonged stimulation by goitrogens such as large doses of iodine for long periods of time. If the swelling is cosmetically unacceptable or is causing pressure symptoms subtotal thyroidectomy is performed.

An *anaplastic carcinoma* of the thyroid presents as a hard multinodular swelling. The voice may be hoarse and the mass fixed to surrounding structures. The prognosis is bleak.

There is a Diffuse Enlargement of the Whole Gland

This occurs in *Grave's Disease*, an autoimmune disease which is the usual cause of thyrotoxicosis (the other cause is a functioning solitary adenoma). Diffuse thyroid swelling may also occur in pregnancy or in puberty but the patient will be found to be euthyroid. Diffuse swelling of the thyroid may also occur in thyroiditis. Grave's Disease is usually treated medically by blocking the effects of thyroxine. Alternatives include ablation of the gland with radioactive iodine or subtotal thyroidectomy.

SWELLINGS OF THE SALIVARY GLANDS

The salivary glands of surgical importance are the parotid gland and the submandibular gland. The swellings are of three types:

Infective

Acute viral (mumps) and bacterial illness can affect the parotid gland and less commonly, the submandibular gland. Acute suppuritive parotitis occurs in dehydrated ill patients and treatment is by rehydration, antibiotics and proper mouth hygiene.

Obstructive

The salivary glands may be blocked by calculi. These are composed of the same material as that which forms scale on the teeth. The submandibular gland is particularly prone to form quite large calculi which block its duct and cause pain on eating. Infection may also supervene. If the stone is located distally in the duct it can be removed locally through the floor of the mouth, other wise the whole gland must be removed. Fine calculi may occur in the parotid but these are uncommon.

Neoplastic

The commonest tumour (65%) occurring in the parotid gland is a pleomorphic adenoma (mixed parotid tumour). It is a slow growing adenoma with an incomplete capsule. Small protrusions of tumour through its capsule prevent its removal by enucleation. Hence it is removed by the operation of superficial parotidectomy. Pleomorphic adenomas are uncommon in the submandibular gland.

Malignant

The presence of a rapidly enlarging swelling, pain and large lymph nodes with facial nerve paralysis suggests that the parotid swelling is malignant. Twenty five percent of parotid tumours are malignant and the figure is higher in the submandibular gland. The most common malignant tumour is a *muco-epidermoid* tumour. *Adenocarcinomas* and *adenoid cystic carcinomas* may also occur. Treatment is total parotidectomy with removal of involved lymph nodes.

OTHER SWELLINGS OF THE NECK

Thyroglossal Cyst

The thyroid gland develops from the lower portion of the thyroglossal duct which begins at the foramen caecum at the back of the tongue. If a portion of this duct remains patent it can form a cyst - thryroglossal cyst. They are commonly found in two sites - between the isthmus of the thyroid gland and the hyoid cartilage and just above the hyoid cartilage. Since they are attached to the base of the tongue, they move when the tongue is protruded. They should be removed for infection is common.

Branchial Cyst

These are thought to be remnants of the first or second branchial pouch. They present as painless swellings which protrude from behind the anterior edge of the upper third of the sternomastoid muscle. Since lymphoid tissue in the cyst wall may become infected surgical removal is usually recommended.

Cystic Hygroma (Lymph Cyst)

These are congenital lymphangiomas which are usually found in the subcutaneous tissues at the base of the posterior triangle of the neck. They may reach a huge size and cause respiratory embarrassment.

Pharyngeal Diverticulum

This is caused by herniation of pharyngeal mucosa through a weak area in the inferior pharyngeal constrictor muscle secondary to cricopharyngeal discoordination. The patient complains of dysphagia, regurgitation of food, chronic cough and recurrent aspiration pneumonia. Malnutrition may be intense. A swelling occasionally is noted in the neck and pressure on it causes gurgling sounds and regurgitation. A barium swallow confirms the diagnosis. Removal of the diverticulum and division of the cricopharyngeal muscle results in total resolution of the problem.

Swellings of Cervical Lymphnodes

Acute Adenitis

Infections of the head and neck may lead to acute lymphadenitis. These are firm tender nodes that decrease in size when infection is resolved.

Chronic Adenitis

These may be secondary to tuberculosis, sarcoidosis or glandular fever. Tuberculosis of the neck glands should not be forgotten. The patient complains of a lump in the neck that may or may not be painful. Examination reveals enlarged nodes matted together. The nodes may coalesce, liquify and turn into a 'cold abscess'. This may burst through the deep cervical fascia and 'point' on the skin (Collar stud abscess). Diagnosis is by biopsy and treatment is by chemotherapy.

Reticulosis

Lymphoma, lymposarcoma and reticulosarcoma present as painless lumps in the neck which grow slowly. Malaise, weight loss and pallor are common symptoms. Biopsy confirms the diagnosis.

Metastases to Lymphnodes

Metastatic deposits of cancer cells in the cervical lymph nodes are the commonest cause of cervical lymphadenopathy in adults. The primary cancer is most often in the upper aero-digestive tract but every possible site must be examined. In 15% of cases the primary cancer is below the clavicles and in 5% the primary is occult. These swellings grow slowly and new swellings may appear. Fine needle aspiration of the nodes is performed and the collected cells sent for cytological examination. This confirms the diagnosis of malignancy. The cancer can then be staged in order to classify the tumour, estimate the prognosis and plan treatment.

FURTHER READING FOR INTEREST

Way, L.W.: Current Surgical Diagnosis and Treatment, 8th Edition, 1988. Appleton and Lange. Pp 224-239

FURTHER READING FOR FINALS

Way, L.W.: Current Surgical Diagnosis and Treatment, 8th Edition, 1988. Appleton and Lange. Pp 240-257

NOTES

Tutorial 9

Carcinoma of the Breast

Breast cancer is the most common neoplasm in women and a leading cause of death in the 35-55 age group. In western societies any individual woman in her lifetime stands a 1-11 to 1-14 chance of developing the disease, the incidence of which is increasing worldwide ranging from 0.2% to 8% per annum.

In some countries of low incidence, such as Japan and Singapore, the rise has so far been observed predominantly in women under the age of 50 and appears to be a birth cohort or generation effect. Such increases are likely to persist throughout life, implying the major increases in breast cancer incidence will occur in such countries 20-30 years from now.

RISK FACTORS

Genetic, Menstrual and Reproductive Factors

The increased risk of breast cancer in first-degree relatives of women who have breast cancer (sisters or daughters) is well recognised. The importance of menstrual and reproductive factors is also clearly established and the increased risk associated with early menarche, late age at menopause, late age at first birth and nulliparity highlights the importance of oestrogenic activity in the aetiology of breast cancer.

Benign Breast Disease

It has generally been accepted that women who have had a previous breast biopsy have a 2-3 fold increased risk of breast cancer. More recently long-term follow up of such patients has established that the risk is largely restricted to the 4% who show atypical hyperplasia, who have a 4 fold increase.

NATURAL HISTOLOGY AND BIOLOGY

Murine studies have established that it takes about 10^9 cancer cells, and 30 population doublings, to produce a 1 cm lesion in humans which is about the smallest clinically discernable mass. Doubling time of human breast cancer is variable but there is evidence that the mean doubling time of early breast cancer is 25 days whereas advanced breast cancer has a mean doubling time of 129 days. The difference is statistically significant and provides convincing evidence for growth retardation in more advanced disease: the so-called Gompertzian pattern.

It will be appreciated that a 1 cm tumour, although clinically early, is biologically late. This accords with recently published data on the long-term 30 year follow up of women with breast cancer which indicates that statistical cure (the attainment of a group subject only to normal mortality risks) has not yet been demonstrated in this disease. Even so, perhaps 25% of women wil experience personal "cure" in that they live without overt signs of their breast cancer until they die from some other cause.

Biologically, breast cancer is almost certainly a systemic disease from early in its life cycle and axillary lymph node involvement is a reflection of a host-tumour relationship that permits development of metastasis rather than being the instigator of distant disease as proposed in the classical hypothesis of sequential stepwise spread from the primary tumour.

These new biological concepts have very important implications for modern approaches to treatment.

PATHOLOGY

Most breast cancers are adenocarcinomas arising from the ductal or lobular epithelium of the terminal ducto-lobular unit. 80% are ductal in type and 9% lobular; the remainder comprising a variety of rare histologic types.

PRESENTATION AND DIAGNOSIS OF BREAST CANCER

The traditional presentation of breast cancer as a palpable lump discovered accidentally has been modified by the widespread use of screening mammography in asymptomatic women and perhaps, to a lesser extent, by breast self-examination.

Breast Cancer Presenting as a Palpable Lump

Most lumps in the breasts are benign and due to complex hormonal interactions on the fibroglandular stroma. *The classical signs suggesting malignancy, however, are easy palpability with the flat of the hand, a firm to hard consistency and surface irregularity.* Skin attachment due to contraction of the suspensory ligaments which pass from the breast cancer to the dermis, is a very important physical sign which may only be apparent on symmetrical inspection during straight arm raising. Inversion of the nipple of recent onset or attachment to the pectoral fascia are less frequent but important features. More advanced disease may show peau d'orange due to lymphatic infiltrations and oedema of the overlying skin and some aggressive tumours present with inflammatory features which fail to respond to antibiotic therapy.

Although the clinical interpretation of axillary nodal involvement has low sensitivity and specificity (with a 30% error both ways), examination of the breast must be completed by careful palpation of the axilla as an important component of clinical staging.

Histologic confirmation of malignancy is essential prior to definitive surgery. Although this can be determined by frozen section examination at the time of operation, it does restrict the opportunity for full discussion with the patient of the options which are now available for breast cancer management. Diagnosis in the out-patient clinic by fine-needle aspiration cytology, or true-cut biopsy, is an important advance in management as it can mean that women are not subjected to the psychological trauma of an anaesthetic uncertain as to whether they will awake with or without a breast.

Breast Cancer Detected by Mammography Screening

Well conducted trials in the United States, Scandinavia and Holland have clearly shown that breast cancer screening by mammography, through early detection of less advanced disease, can lower mortality in women over 50 years of age by as much as 30%. Technical advances have not only strikingly improved the quality of the x-ray image but also reduced the dose of radiation so that outside screening trials increasing numbers of asymptomatic women are now being referred by their primary doctors to Radiology Centres equipped with facilities for film screen mammography. Mammographically breast cancer may present as circumscribed or stellate lesions, microcalficiations or thickening of the skin of the breast due to lymphoedema. Each presents varying problems of perception and analysis and experience is required for accurate interpretation.

Many of these lesions are impalpable and their detection has required the development of hook wire and/or dye marker techniques as a guide to surgical localisation and biopsy.

Distant Metastases

Patients with confirmed breast cancer should be carefully examined for evidence of distant metastases. Some breast cancers have a particular biologic propensity to metastasise to viscera; others spread to bone. Chest x-ray should be a routine investigation and any disturbance of liver biochemistry, particularly elevation of alkaline phosphatase, is an indication for assessment of the liver by upper abdominal ultrasound. Skeletal scintigraphy is useful as a base-line study but it does not affect the choice of primary surgery and may be deferred until the postoperative period. Further scanning is not recommended in the absence of symptoms.

Staging

1982-International Union against Cancer (UICC) T N M classification, where the system is used to convey information obtained after surgery.

- p T1: Tumour of 2 cm or less in its greatest dimension
- p T2: >2 cm but not more than 5 cm
- p T3: >5 cm
- p T4: Tumour of any size with direct extension to chest wall or skin

Regional Lymph Nodes (p N)

- p N0: No evidence of invasion of regional nodes
- p N1: Evidence of invasion of "movable" homolateral axillary lymph nodes
- p N2: Evidence of invasion of homolateral axillary lymph nodes fixed to one another or to other structures
- p N3: Evidence of invasion of homolateral supraclavicular or infraclavicular nodes

Distant Metastases (M)

- M0: No evidence of distant metastases
- M1: Distant metastases present, including skin involvement beyond the breast area.

PRIMARY TREATMENT OF OPERABLE BREAST CANCER

New understanding of the biological nature of breast cancer has dramatically altered our perception of the role of surgery in the management. Very long-term follow up of the B-04 trial conducted in the early 1970's in the United States and Canada has confirmed that radical-en-bloc surgery does not influence survival when compared to simple mastectomy. Instead modern surgery is based upon the twin principles of local control of disease and determination of the status of the axiliary lymph nodes.

Not because the regional nodes act as a source of tertiary spread to the skeleton and vital organs but for the reason that their status is the best prognostic guide which is freely available. Two surgical options may be considered.

Less than Mastectomy

In women with primary breast tumours up to 4 cms in size less than mastectomy, combined with axillary dissection, has a disease free and overall survival which is not statistically different from more radical operations involving total removal of the breast. Radiotherapy to the breast only is recommended following local excision for although it does not affect survival it does significantly reduce the local recurrence rate, particularly in patients with positive axillary nodes.

Total Mastectomy

The Patey, or modified radical mastectomy, was introduced in the 1950's as a muscle conserving alternative to the classical radical en-bloc operation in which mastectomy was combined with total axillary lymph node clearance following removal of the overlying pectoral muscles, major and minor.

Although the modified radical mastectomy gives excellent local control, breast cancer staging can be as accurately achieved with less morbidity by restricting the axillary clearance to the nodes contained in the lower third below the lower border of pectoralis minor.

During the past decade there has been an increasing awareness of the serious emotional consequences which may be associated with loss of the female breast. Less than mastectomy may be appropriate for selected women, but largely because of the requirement for radiotherapy, it is not always the alternative of choice. For this reason immediate or delayed breast reconstruction using artificial prostheses, or tissue flaps from latissimus dorsi or rectus abdominus, may prove to be an advance in management.

Prognostic Indices

<u>Axillary Lymph Nodes</u>

The status of the axillary lymph nodes in operable breast cancer patients remains the most important guide to prognosis and it has been demonstrated that if 4 or more nodes are involved with tumour, less than 20% of patients survive 10 years. The outlook for node negative patients is strikingly better but even in this better prognosis group 20-30% of such patients have died or show recurrence of disease at 10 years.

Receptors

In 1896 Beatson demonstrated striking tumour regression following oophorectomy in young women with advanced breast cancer, but it was not until the 1960's, when tritiated estrogens of high specific activity became available, that some understanding of the mechanisms involved in the endocrine response began to emerge. It is now known that many breast cancers possess nuclear receptors (ER) capable of binding oestradiol and that 60% of cancers with this capacity respond to endocrine manipulation. The progesterone receptor (PR) is initiated by the oestrogenic stimulation of ER and their presence improves the predicted accuracy for hormonal responsiveness to 70-75%.

In primary breast cancer the presence of receptors has positive prognostic significance in node positive patients but those who are ER negative are at a greater risk of recurrence. The same trend is suggested in node negative subsets but has not as yet been unequivocably confirmed.

Other Indices

Tumour size and histologic grade are also important risk factors and there are a number of promising new indices such as the pattern of DNA distribution, the percentage of cells in S phase and the expression of the oncogene Her-2/Neu which may enable high risk groups, particularly those with negative nodes to be identified with much greater accuracy.

ADJUVANT THERAPY

The biologic hypothesis that breast cancer is a systemic disease from an early stage in its life cycle supports the arguments for the use of systemic anti-cancer therapy adjuvant to surgery. Analysis of numerous well conducted randomised prospective trials carried out over the past 20 years provides indisputable evidence that chemotherapy substantially prolongs disease-free and overall survivial among pre-menopausal patients. The survival difference between treated and untreated patients is 10-25% at the point of maximum follow-up giving 3-5 additional years of life for treated pre-menopausal women.

The anti-oestrogen drug tamoxifen, introduced in the mid-1970's, has also been extensively tested in an adjuvant setting. In an analysis of 28 trials involving over

16,000 women there was a clear reduction in mortality only among women aged 50 or older in whom tamoxifen reduced the annual odds of death during the first 5 years by about one-fifth.

The field of adjuvant therapy for patients with operable breast cancer, including those with negative axillary nodes, is complex and evolving. Many new questions are being addressed in current prospective trials and there is guarded optimism that significant improved survival will be achieved over the next two decades until a more fundamental approach to cancer is achieved through advances in molecular biology and gene stabilisation.

ADVANCED BREAST CANCER

Tamoxifen

The anti-oestrogen tamoxifen is widely used as a first-line therapy for the treatment of metastatic breast cancer. Although only 30% of patients achieve an objective response at least 50% benefit in terms of disease stabilisation and symptom control.

Tamoxifen competes with oestradiol for the ER binding site and inhibits cell growth in the G1 phase of the cell cycle. It also has other rather complex actions through the medium of growth factors which either promote or inhibit cell proliferation. Nevertheless the paradox is that approximately 10% of ER negative tumours respond to tamoxifen and for this reason anti-oestrogens tend to be the first treatment option in advanced disease, regardless of the receptor status.

Tamoxifen is generally a very well tolerated drug and in responsive patients it can sustain an excellent quality of life. With evidence of relapse and progressive disease there are a number of other hormonal approaches which may be used prior to the initiation of chemotherapy. Aminoglutethamide is an aromatase inhibitor and in post-menopausal women where oestrogen is predominantly synthesised in adipose tissue it can block the conversion of adrenal androgens to estrogens by the aromatase enzyme.

Progestins have also been used successfully in advanced breast cancer in both pre and post-menopausal women. The mechanism of action is largely unknown but response is more likely in patients who are receptor positive.

Combination Chemotherapy

Combination chemotherapy using 3 or more agents, each with a different mode of action or acting at a different point in the cell cycle, is standard secondline therapy in advanced breast cancer. The combination frequently used is cyclophosphamide given orally between days 1 and 14 and methotrexate and 5-fluorouracyl given intravenously on days 1 and 8. The cycle is then repeated according to tolerance at 28 day intervals.

The response rate of 50-60% achieved by chemotherapy is significantly higher than that obtained with endocrine procedures. Nevertheless, complete follow-up has demonstrated no significant difference in survival which argues persuasively for an initial trial of endocrine therapy in all of those with rapidly progressive disease and particularly when associated with negative receptors.

FURTHER READING FOR INTEREST

Forrest, A.P.M. (1986) Advances in the Management of Carcinoma of the Breast. Surg Gynaecol Obst 163 89

FURTHER READING FOR FINALS

Way, L.W. Current Surgical Diagnosis and Treatment. 8th Edition, 1988 Appleton and Lange. Pp 507, 271-275

NOTES

Tutorial 10

Swellings of the Groin

The most common groin swellings are hernias. A hernia is a protrusion of a sac of peritoneum together with preperitoneal fat through a defect in the abdominal wall. The sac may contain omentum, small bowel, colon (rare) or ovary or testes (very rare). The peritoneal sac may protrude into the inguinal canal (inguinal hernia) or femoral canal (femoral hernia).

SURGICAL ANATOMY

The inguinal canal passes obliquely through the anterior abdominal wall just above the medial half of the inguinal ligament. It extends from the deep inguinal ring at the midpoint of the inguinal ligament to the superficical inguinal ring at the pubic crest. The spermatic cord, comprising the remnants of the processus vaginalis, the vas deferens and their nerves and vessels, enters the inguinal canal through the deep inguinal ring and leaves it to enter the scrotum through the superficial inguinal ring. If a hernial sac protrudes directly forwards into the inguinal canal medial to the inferior epigastric artery this is a Direct Inguinal Hernia. If a hernial sac follows the more indirect route of the processus vaginalis through the deep inguinal ring, into the spermatic cord and out through the superficial inguinal ring, it is an Indirect Inguinal Hernia. The sac of a Femoral Hernia does not pass into the inguinal canal at all. It follows the circuitous route of the femoral canal which passes beneath the most medial aspect of the inguinal ligament into the upper thigh.

APPLIED ANATOMY

The inguinal region on the right side may be examined by the surgeon standing to the patient's right side. The tip of the middle finger of the surgeon's right hand is placed on the pubic tubercle and the rest of the finger is made to lie along the line of the inguinal canal. If the right index and ring fingers are spread apart it will be found that the former lies over the site where a direct inguinal hernia will protrude and the latter lies over the site of a protruding femoral hernia. The middle finger itself, lying along the line of the inguinal canal will feel a cough impulse if the patient has an indirect inguinal hernia. Clearly, pressure over the deep inguinal ring would prevent omentum or small intestine entering an indirect hernial sac when the patient is asked to cough.

SOME DEFINITIONS

Strangulation

This means that the blood supply of the contents of the sac is cut off. If the small bowel is strangulated it is a surgical emergency. The patient will suffer from intestinal obstruction and the bowel may undergo infarction.

Neck of Sack

This is the site where the hernial sac first protrudes through the defect in the abdominal wall. It is a tight ring of peritoneum and is the usual site of strangulation.

Incarceration

Occurs when the contents of the sac are fixed within it either because of their size or adhesions. The hernia cannot be returned to the abdominal cavity but it is not strangulated.

Sliding Hernia

If the colon which is normally extra peritoneal forms one side of the sac it is thought to have slid down the canal pulling the peritoneum with it.

DIFFERENTIAL DIAGNOSIS OF AN INGUINAL HERNIA

A fluid filled cyst of the processus vaginalis may occur - it is called a <u>hydrocele of the cord</u> and can be distinguished from a hernia by the fact that it does not expand when the patient coughs (cough impulse) and it does not disappear (i.e. it is not reducible) when gentle pressure is applied over it. A <u>lipoma of the cord</u> is indistinguishable clinically from a hydrocele of the cord. Both of these inguinal swellings move when the testicle is tugged. If there is not a testis in the scrotum of a patient with an inguinal swelling on the same side the swelling may be an <u>undescended testicle.</u> <u>Ectopic testicles</u> lie superficial to the inguinal canal and are much more easily felt than undescended testicles.

Other Swellings that may occur in the Groin

Enlarged lymph nodes, and femoral artery aneurysms are not difficult to distinguish from hernias. If the patient is standing up a varicosity of the proximal saphenous vein (saphena-varix) may look very like a femoral hernia. Not only does it have a fluid thrill within it when the long saphenous vein in percussed, however, but it also disappears when the patient lies down.

Diagnosis of a Large Inguino- Scrotal Mass

Sometimes a patient will present with a very large scrotal mass and it may be difficult to decide if this is a large indirect hernia which is passing from above into the scrotum or if it is swelling arising from the scrotum itself. The key to diagnosis is for the surgeon to place his hands around the neck of the scrotum and ask the question 'Can I get above this swelling or not?' If not, the swelling is a hernia. Otherwise it will be a large epididymal cyst or a hydrocele. These two conditions can be differentiated by remembering that a hydrocele completely surrounds the testis and only one swelling can be felt in the scrotum. On the other hand, an epididymal cyst is separate from the underlying testes, two swellings can be felt in the scrotum and the patient may think he has a third testicle. In the fourteenth century the Pope granted a petition from a man who wanted to marry two wives because he possessed three testicles.

SOME IMPORTANT POINTS ABOUT GROIN HERNIAS

Indirect Inguinal Hernias

Nearly all inguinal hernias in babies, children and young adults are indirect inguinal hernias. Indirect hernias are probably 'congenital' and although they frequently present in the first year of life the first clinical evidence may not appear until middle or old age when increased intrabdominal pressure and dilatation of the deep inguinal ring allow abdominal contents to enter the previously empty incompletely obliterated processus vaginalis. Although indirect hernias are the most common groin hernias in both sexes, at all ages they have an overwhelming male preponderance. Because indirect hernias lie within the spermatic cord they can, and frequently do, enter the scrotum. Not uncommonly the neck of the sac of an indirect hernia may obstruct the lumen of a loop of small intestine leading to small bowel obstruction with *small bowel colic, vomiting, central abdominal distension and obstipation*. If left untreated, strangulation may occur.

Indirect inguinal hernias should all be treated surgically. Most can have their operation as day cases under general or local anaesthesia. The sac is removed (herniotomy) and the posterior wall of the inguinal canal is repaired (herniorraphy). The best repair is that used at The Shouldice Clinic in Toronto, Canada.

Direct Inguinal Hernias

These hernias are due to an acquired weakness in the abdominal wall. They are exceptional in females and in patients under 40 years of age. Direct hernias virtually never enter the scrotum. Obstruction and strangulation are also rare because these hernias have a wide neck. Treatment is by herniorraphy using the Shouldice technique.

Femoral Hernias

Femoral Hernias are acquired and present below and lateral to the pubic tubercle. They are less common than inguinal hernias in both men and women but are more common in women. They are prone to obstruction and strangulation because of the rigid and unyielding nature of the femoral ring. Thus all patients with a bowel obstruction, particularly those who are obese, should have the area below and lateral to the pubic tubercle palpated carefully in case there is an obstructed femoral hernia present. All femoral hernias require surgical repair because of this danger of obstruction. Repair involves removal of the sac and closure of the femoral canal.

OTHER TYPES OF ABDOMINAL HERNIAS

For completeness three types of abdominal hernias are mentioned here even though they are unrelated to swellings of the groin. They are epigastric, umbilical and hiatus hernias.

Epigastric and Umbilical Hernias

These hernias are considered together because a para-umbilical hernia is an epigastric hernia situated just above the umbilicus. These hernias protrude through a defect in the linea alba between the xiphisternum and umbilicus. Epigastric hernias are usually small but sometimes can be quite painful. Umbilical hernias in adults (paraumbilical) present in obese patients and may become as large as an orange. The chronicity of the condition leads to adhesions within the sac and the contents are frequently irreducible. Obtruction within the sac not infrequently occurs and requires emergency surgery.

Infantile umbilical hernias occur through a persistent defect or incomplete contraction of the umbilical scar. The majority close spontaneously by the end of the first year of life.

Hiatus Hernia

There are two typs of hernia that occur at the oesophageal hiatus. The majority are *sliding hernias* in which the gastro-oesophageal junction slides upwards into the mediastinum. This leads to incompetence of the cardio-oesophageal junction and reflux of gastric contents. Reflux oesophagitis may then occur which may be complicated by chronic blood loss and stricture formation.

Para-oesophageal hernias occur occasionally, usually in the elderly. Here the fundus of the stomach rotates in front of the oesophagus and herniates through the hiatus into the mediastinum inside a large hernial sac. Although many patients with sliding hernias which are causing symptoms can be treated conservatively (weight loss, elevation of bed and H2 blockers) and only a few need surgical repair (Nissen Fundoplication). Most patients with para oesophageal hernias should have surgical reduction of the hernia and repair of the diaphragm because of the risk of stomach strangulation.

FURTHER READING FOR INTEREST

Devlin H.B. et al (1986): Short Day Surgery for Inguinal Hernia: Experience of the Shouldice Operation 1970-1982. Br J Surg 73, 123

Kirk, R.M. (1983) : Which Inguinal Hernia Repair? Br Med J 287, 4

FURTHER READING FOR FINALS

Way, L.W. : Current Surgical Diagnosis and Treatment. 8th Edition, 1988 Appleton and Lange , Pp 649-660, 385-389

Browse, N.(1978): An Introduction to the Symptoms and Signs of Surgical Disease. Edward Arnold, London. Pp 310-322

NOTES

Tutorial 11

Trauma

Trauma in New Zealand, as in other developed societies, has become the leading cause of death in the first four decades of life. It accounts for more than 1700 deaths and over 60,000 hospital admissions per year in this country. You will commonly see patients on surgical wards who have sustained injuries of various types.

CLASSIFICATION

Trauma is generally categorised by both the mechanism of injury, and the body region affected.

Mechanism of Injury

Blunt trauma is the most common mechanism of injury and may occur as a result of road crashes, falls or assaults.
Penetrating trauma is uncommon in New Zealand and describes gunshot, shotgun and stab wounds.

Body Region

For descriptive purposes the body is divided into six body regions.

> Head Region
> Face Region
> Thorax Region
> Abdomen Region
> Extremities Region
> External Region

Multiple trauma, such as often occurs in road crashes, results in injuries in more than one body region.

CLINICAL PRESENTATION

Unlike other conditions trauma does not lend itself to the taking of a detailed history, followed by clinical examination, investigations and subsequent treatment. Initial assessment of the patient must follow a sequence of priorities with life threatening injuries being treated as they are recognised.

Primary Survey

A - Airway

Provision or maintenance of an airway has the highest priority as an inadequate airway can kill within minutes. Unconscious patients do not maintain an adequate airway. In patients suffering blunt trauma specific consideration should be given to the *possibility of cervical spine injury* and the patient's neck should not be hyperflexed to establish or maintain an airway.

B - Breathing

Airway patency does not ensure adequate ventilation. Adequate air exchange, in addition to an open airway, is required. This can be established using the basic principles of *look, feel and listen*. Two traumatic conditions that most often compromise ventilation are *tension pneumothorax, and large flail chest with pulmonary contusion*.

C - Circulation

All traumatic conditions are associated with haemorrhage which is a prominent, treatable cause of early post-injury death. Rapid and accurate assessment of the injured patient's haemodynamic status is therefore essential. Three elements of observation yield key information within seconds. These are *state of consciousness, skin colour and pulse*. When blood volume is reduced by half or more cerebral perfusion is critically impaired and unconsciousness results. The ashen grey skin of the face and the white skin of blood drained extremities implies at least loss of 30% of blood volume.

Significant haemorrhage usually occurs in one or more of the following areas.

External haemorrhage results from external wounds and is easily identified and controlled by direct pressure.

Internal haemorrhage results when bleeding occurs into one of the body cavities. Bleeding in the chest is called a haemothorax and up to 2 litres of blood (40% of blood volume) may accumulate in a single thoracic activity. Bleeding in the abdomen is called a *haemoperitoneum* and may result from any injury to an intra-abdominal organ. Most commonly the solid organs (liver, spleen and kidneys)are injured in blunt trauma. Significant bleeding also occurs in association with fractures. A single fractured femur may result in loss of up to 1.5 litres of blood into the thigh muscle and a fractured pelvis may exsanguinate the patient.

D - Disability

A brief neurological examiniation should be performed at this stage comprising an assessment of the patient's *level of consciousness and pupillary size and reaction*. Level of consciousness can simply be assessed using the AVPU mnemonic:

    A - Awake and Alert
    V - responds to Verbal Stimuli
    P - responds to Painful Stimuli
    U - Unconscious

Patients who are initially awake and alert and subsequently have a deterioration in their level of consciousness are particularly likely to have intracranial collections of blood *(extradural and subdural haematomas)* which are amenable to surgical evacuation.

E - Exposure

If not already completed the patient must be *undressed* at this stage so that a complete examiniation can be undertaken.

Resuscitation

Airway maintenance, cardiopulmonary resuscitation and other life-saving modalities must be initiated as the problems are identified. Resuscitation of the ABCs must continue with priority over other diagnostic and therapeutic considerations. Essential diagnostic X-rays (lateral cervical spine X-ray, chest X-ray, pelvic X-ray) should be undertaken and monitoring devices (ECG, nasogastric tube, urinary catheter) placed during this phase. *Only when resuscitation has resulted in a stable or stabilising patient should further evaluation be undertaken.*

Secondary Survey

The secondary survey is a complete head-to-toe, front to back examination that aims to identify all injuries.

Head

The secondary survey begins with an examination of the head region. The entire scalp should be palpated for lacerations and fractures, the mastoid area inspected for evidence of a *Battles sign* and the ears examined for *haemotympanum*. Both these signs are evidence of a basal skull fracture. The eyes should be re-evaluated for pupillary size, and fundi for haemorrhages. A more complete assessment of the level of consciousness should be undertaken at this point using the *Glasgow Coma Scale*.

The neck should be both visually inspected and palpated. *The absence of neurological deficit, pain, or tenderness does not rule out injury to the cervical spine.* Such an injury should be presumed to be present until ruled out by adequate radiological examination.

Face

The entire face should be palpated for evidence of fractures. Maxillo-facial trauma not associated with airway obstruction, however, should only be treated after the patient is completely stabilised.

Thorax

A complete examination of the chest requires visual examination, palpation of the entire chest cage, and auscultation. Contusions and haematomas of the chest wall are often signs of more serious occult injury. Pneumothorax and haemothorax are common in trauma to the chest region.

Abdomen

Any abdominal injury is potentially life threatening, but the specific diagnosis is not as important as establishing that an abdominal injury exists. *Clinical examination (look, feel and listen) is unreliable in those who have suffered a head injury or who are intoxicated by drugs or alcohol.* In these patients other forms of abdominal assessment are required such as diagnostic peritoneal lavage or abdominal CT scanning. Rectal examination, however, is an important part of the abdominal evaluation as it will detect the presence of blood within the bowel, a high-riding prostate, the presence of pelvic fractures, the integrity of the rectal wall, and the quality of sphincter tone.

Extremities

The extremities must be examined visually for evidence of injury and then functionally. If the patient is awake and co-operative active range of motion should be sought in each limb.

External

Examination of the entire integument, including the back, should be undertaken. All trauma patients have external injuries which may be signs of more severe internal injuries.

HISTORY

A history of the mechanisms of injury is very helpful in identifying potential injuries suffered by the patient. In general, the severity of injury is proportional to the *amount of energy transferred* from an object to the human body. *Direction of energy transfer* is also important. With this information *it is possible to predict injury patterns* that may be suffered by that patient. An example would be the rapid frontal deceleration which occurs when a car collides head on with a bridge abutment. The pattern of injuries suffered by a restrained patient might include a closed head injury, flail chest, thoracic aortic rupture and fracture of the pelvis.

In penetrating trauma the type of injury is determined by the region of the body sustaining injury and the transfer of energy from the projectile to the body. In gunshot wounds this transfer of energy is related to the mass and velocity of the bullet.

Limited pertinent past medical history is usually available in these patients. Particularly relevant facts, if obtainable, may be remembered by the mnemonic AMPLE:

    A- Allergies
    M- Medications
    P- Past Illness
    L- Last Meal
    E- Events surrounding injury

RECORDS

Trauma evaluation is a dynamic process with the patient's status often changing rapidly. In addition, multiple specialties and doctors are often involved with the overall care of the patient changing from one team to another. For these, as well as medico-legal reasons, meticulous record keeping is essential.

SUMMARY

The injured patient must be evaluated rapidly with life threatening injuries being identified and treated at the same time. Once established, a thorough 'head-to-toe' examination is required to identify all injuries. History of the mechanism of injury is crucial to the assessment as it may be the only clue to the likely injuries the patient has suffered.

FURTHER READING FOR INTEREST

Way, L.W.: Current Surgical Diagnosis and Treatment. 8th Edition, 1988. Appleton and Lange   Pp 187-208

FURTHER READING FOR FINALS

Way, L.W.: Current Surgical Diagnosis and Treatment. 8th Edition, 1988. Appleton and Lange   Pp 210-216

NOTES

Tutorial 12

Peripheral Vascular Disease

Peripheral vascular disease is a degenerative process resulting from atherosclerosis affecting the arterial tree. It is so common that it could be regarded as universally present in the elderly but not all patients are so affected as to be symptomatic. Predisposing causes include *smoking, diabetes mellitus, and hyperlipidaemias*.

PATTERNS OF DISEASE

As a result of the buildup of cholesterol plaque in the arterial wall and the breakdown of its anatomic integrity one of two common patterns of disease emerge. Where the prodominant feature is the laying down of cholesterol containing plaque the arterial tree becomes blocked, so called *occlusive* vascular disease. Where the predominant feature is degeneration of the arterial wall, a dilatation of the artery occurs, forming an *aneurysm*.

MECHANISM OF SYMPTOMS

Whether the pattern is occlusive or aneurysmal arterial disease causes symptoms as a result of three mechanisms, *obstruction* when the artery becomes blocked, *embolism* when blood clot, platelet thrombus or cholesterol debris from the lining of the artery are taken distally by the blood flow and block smaller arteries, or *rupture* where a weakened artery bursts.

ANATOMIC SITES

While any area of the peripheral arterial tree may be affected by atherosclerosis the three most common areas affected are the *extracranial carotid system*, the *aortoiliac system* and the *femoropopliteal system*.

INVESTIGATIONS

Investigations of the peripheral vascular system may be either *invasive* or *non-invasive*. Non-invasive tests are those which do not require any instrumentation of the patient's body but merely the placement of instruments on the outside to obtain readings of some type. The two most common non-invasive investigations of the peripheral vascular system are *duplex ultrasound* and *computerised tomography*.

Invasive tests refer to those in which catheters are placed in the arterial system and contrast material injected. The most common invasive test is called an *angiogram*.

EXTRACRANIAL CAROTID DISEASE

The pattern of disease most often found in this site is occlusive, with aneurysm being rare. The mechanism of production of symptoms is either occlusive or embolic. As is common with atherosclerosis the precise site affected involves a bifurcation and in this region it is the point where the internal and external carotid arteries arise from the common carotid.

Symptoms

Occlusive vascular disease in the carotid system produces symptoms as a result of distal ischaemia. These may be:

> *Stroke* - a permanent neurologic deficit resulting from occlusion of a major intracerebral artery.
>
> *Reversible Ischaemic Neurological Deficit (RIND)* - A "stroke" that resolves completely after more than 1 but less than 24 hours. This is usually caused by an embolism of either platelet thrombus or cholesterol debris that breaks up after a period of time with subsequent return of blood flow.
>
> *Transient Ischaemic Attack (TIA)* - a "stroke" that lasts usually a few minutes to an hour and resolves without deficit. The cause is usually embolic.
>
> *Amaurosis Fugax (AF)* - a transient ischaemic attack affecting the blood supply to the eye. The sufferer notes a loss of vision in one eye, usually coming down like a curtain over the upper half of the visual field and lasting for some minutes.

Investigations

Duplex ultrasound is used to determine the haemodynamic significance of any obstruction to the extracranial carotid system. A stenosis over 80% of the cross-sectional area of an artery is regarded as significant. While duplex ultrasound is a good investigation for determining stenosis it may not pick up the irregularities in the wall of the artery which may be the cause of emboli, commonly implicated in cerebral ischaemic events.

Angiography is usually performed after placing a catheter in a groin artery and advancing it to the common carotid artery. Radiographic contrast material is injected and a map of the arteries in the neck obtained, either with regular X-ray plates or on a computer screen using a technique known as digital subtraction. Angiography caries a small risk of stroke or TIA (0.1%) but gives the most complete information on the arterial system.

Treatment

Symptomatic extracranial carotid vascular disease may be treated either medically, using agents that stop platelet aggregation such as aspirin, or surgically by removing the buildup of cholesterol plaque inside the carotid artery.

Medical treatment with aspirin reduces the overall risk of stroke 25% and does not expose the patient to the risks of an operation.

Surgical treatment is called endarterectomy (removal of the lining of the carotid artery). This operation has a combined risk of stroke or death of 3% but if successful reduces the risk of subsequent stroke by 80%.

The decision about whether patients should be treated medically or surgically is a complex one and relates to the individual patient's risk of stroke, their fitness for surgery, and the capability of the surgeon to perform a successful operation.

AORTOILIAC DISEASE

Both aneurysmal and occlusive patterns of disease are found in this site. In aneurysmal disease symptoms are predominantly produced by rupture although embolism occasionally occurs. In occlusive disease obstruction to blood flow is the predominant cause for symptoms.

Aneurysms

Aneurysms affect the aorta and iliac arteries and are likely to cause symptoms when they reach 2-3 times the size of the original artery .

<u>Symptoms</u>

Most aneurysms are *asymptomatic* and are diagnosed incidentally during physical examination or during investigation for some other condition (such as when a patient undergoes ultrasound examination for gallstones). When rupture is imminent, aneurysms may produce symptoms of back and left flank pain and following rupture these symptoms are associated with profound shock.

Investigations

Ultrasound examination is usually sufficient to diagnose the presence of an aneurysm and show its size and extent. If there is clinical evidence of impairment of renal function, or if lower extremity pulses are not normal it may be necessary to perform *angiography* to demonstrate the nature and extent of associated occlusive disease. Occasionally, when there is concern that the aneurysm may extend proximal to the origin of the renal arteries (a suprarenal aneurysm) CT may be required to show the exact extent.

Treatment

Once an aneurysm has enlarged to a size where risk of rupture exists (4 cm in the abdominal aorta) *surgical repair* is indicated. Mortality after emergency repair of a ruptured aortic aneurysm approaches 50% whereas that for elective repair is less than 5%. The weakened section of artery is replaced with a segment of a knitted dacron tube sutured above and below to the normal artery. If the iliac arteries are also aneurysmal a bifurcated graft is used to replace the entire aorto-iliac segment.

Occlusive Disease

Symptoms

Occlusive disease of the lower extremities results in not enough blood flow reaching the lower legs. This may cause one or more of the following symptoms:

Claudication
This is a tight pain not unlike that described in the chest region in myocardial ischaemia. It most commonly affects the calf muscles but may also affect the thigh and buttock region. It is predictable, in that it comes on after a set period of exercise and resolves after a period of rest. Claudication may be disabling if a patient's employment or quality of life is affected but it is not life threatening.

Rest pain
In more severe ischaemia patients may suffer rest pain. This affects the foot, usually under the toes and metatarsal region and occurs when the patient is at rest in the horizontal position (such as in bed at night). The lack of gravity assistance to flow results in critical ischaemia and patients classically go to sleep at night and wake

after 2-3 hours with pain in the foot which is relieved when they hang the foot out of bed. This symptom is indicative of limb threatening ischaemia.

Ulcers

Ischaemic ulcers occur either on the foot or the lateral aspect of the ankle and are also a sign of critical limb threatening ischaemia.

Gangrene

The most severe presentation of distal ischaemia is that of gangrene where tissue death has occurred.

Investigations

In patients with disabling claudication or limb threatening symtoms, angiography is indicated to delineate the nature of the occlusions and stenoses.

Treatment

Depending on the arteriographic findings either surgery or angioplasty may be indicated. In narrowest areas (stenoses) or short occlusions, particularly in the iliac system angioplasty is appropriate. This procedure is performed by the radiologist who passes a guidewire across the stenosis or occlusion and then passes a balloon tipped catheter over the guidewire. When the balloon is inflated the atheromatous plaque is split and squeezed out of the lumen. In extensive occlusions this procedure is not possible and surgical bypass is indicated. Usually this involves placement of a bifurcated knitted dacron tube graft from the aorta to the common femoral artery, bypassing the obstruction.

Femoropopliteal Disease

The most common pattern of disease in this region is occlusive but aneurysms may also be present, particularly if the patient has aortoiliac aneurysm disease. Either way the mechanism of production of symptoms is usually obstructive.

Aneurysms

Symptoms

In this region aneurysms either occlude or embolise distally and seldom rupture. They may be present in either the common femoral or popliteal arteries. They usually present with symptoms related to distal ischaemia as outlined above and are seldom discovered incidentally unless the patient is being evaluated for an aortic or contralateral lower extremity aneurysm.

Investigations

While *ultrasound* is usually adequate to diagnose the size and extent of the aneurysm the nature of the surgical reconstruction requires that *angiography* be undertaken to define the full vascular anatomy.

Treatment

The risks of occlusion and embolisation associated with lower extremity aneurysms demands their repair regardless of size. In the common femoral region the most common approach is to replace the artery with a small segment of an artificial graft material after excising the aneurysm. In the popliteal region the artery is less accessible and it is more common to bypass the artery from above the knee to below the knee and then exclude it from the arterial flow.

Occlusive Disease

The most common site affected by occlusive disease is the femoral artery in the adductor canal immediately above the knee.

Symptoms

Occlusive lower extremity vascular disease may be associated with *claudication, rest pain, ulcers* or *gangrene*. Patients with disabling claudication or limb threatening symptoms merit investigation.

Investigations

Angiography is required to delineate the vascular anatomy.

Treatment

Depending on the anatomy of the occlusions either *angioplasty* or *surgical bypass* may be indicated. The more distal the occlusion (closer to the foot) the more difficult both therapies become. In general angioplasty is indicated for stenoses and short occlusions (<10 cm) above the knee. For longer occlusions or disease below the knee surgical bypass is indicated. Bypass is preferably performed using the patient's own saphenous vein, either in a reversed fashion (to prevent the valves stopping flow) or in-situ after destruction of the valves. If a suitable vein is not available bypass has to be performed with an artificial graft usually expanded polytetrafluoroethylene (PTFE).

Occasionally when these approaches have not been possible or have been unsuccessful it is possible to attempt to increase skin blood flow via lumbar sympathectomy. In this procedure the sympathetic chain responsible for autonomic inflow to the skin of the region is blocked by injecting phenol around the sympathetic chain after passing a needle percutaneously. This is occasionally helpful in situations of rest pain, ulcers or limited gangrene.

FURTHER READING FOR INTEREST

Way, L.W.: Current Surgical Diagnosis and Treatment. 8th Edition, 1988 Appleton and Lange Pp 674-703

FURTHER READING FOR FINALS

Nil

NOTES

Tutorial 13

Diseases of the Venous System

VENOUS ULCERS

Most leg ulcers are due to venous hypertension but remember that a significant minority are due to other causes.

Pathology

The essential element in chronic ulceration is ischaemia at the level of the microcirculation. Although the arterial supply of the limb as assessed by foot pulses may be adequate the ulcer refuses to heal because of ischaemia of the skin cells. In venous hypertension the cellular ischaemia is due to 2 factors, capillary stasis and oedema.

The pathophysiology is best understood by considering the venous haemodynamics in the normal lower limb. The superficial veins of the limb are in the subcutaneous fat. They communicate with the deep veins via the perforating (communicating) veins. There are many valves in the superficial and deep veins, increasing in frequency from above downwards. In less than 20% of people there is a valve above the groin level. The valves in the superficial and deep veins only allow flow in a cephalad direction. The valves in the perforating veins only allow flow from superficial to deep. The deep veins of the limb are surrounded by muscle. In the calf the muscle is surrounded by a dense, virtually unstretchable, membrane - the investing deep fascia. When the muscles relax the blood is prevented from refluxing by the venous valves. This results in a relative vacuum in the deep compartment to be pumped up towards the heart and the pressure in the superficial veins is kept low. This is the mechanism of the calf muscle pump.

If the valves in the superficial veins are defective, as they are in patients with varicose veins, blood will reflux from the deep to the superficial system, most commonly at the junction of the saphenous and femoral veins in the groin. This increases the pressure in the superficial veins. If the valves in the short saphenous or perforating veins are incompetent the same thing happens. If the valves in the deep veins are incompetent, blood will reflux in the deep veins between muscle contractions. The effects of an increase in venous pressure in either system is transmitted to the venous end of the capillary loop. This back pressure will result in reduction or abolition of flow in the capillary loop. It will also result in oedema. Because the hydrostatic pressure at the venous end of the capillary loop exceeds the osmotic pressure within the loop, tissue fluid will not be reabsorbed so will remain as oedema. Because of the high pressure within the loop, whole blood extravasates, increasing the protein content of the tissue fluid and thus reducing further the osmotic pull of the intravascular fluid on the extra vascular fluid. Blood pigments and fibrin will collect in the tissues. Because of the reduction in capillary flow there wil be relative ischaemia of the cells of the skin. This will be compounded by the oedema. Oedema, whatever its cause, shifts cells further from their capillary of supply thus reducing the gradient for diffusion of nutrients and metabolites.

Clinical Picture

Symptoms
It is often said that venous ulcers are not painful. This is not true. They are often painful but the pain can always be abolished by giving appropriate antibiotics systemically.

Physical Signs
Venous ulcers occur most frequently on the medial side of the limb above or about the medial malleolus. They can, however, occur anywhere in the lower leg or on the foot. They are shallow and do not go deeper than the deep fascia. There may be surrounding cellulitis. The edges are relatively flat but this varies according to the amount of oedema present.

There are 3 cardinal signs of venous ulceration - *oedema, dry eczema and pigmentation*. If these are not present the ulcer is not venous in origin. Sometimes there may be a wet eczema. This will be due to allergy to some preparation which has been put on the ulcer. Allergies are common in this group of patients for they have often had numerous chemicals applied to the area in attempts to produce healing.

Differential Diagnosis

It must be remembered that venous hypertension is common and that non venous ulcers may occur in patients who have signs of venous hypertension. Squamous and basal cell carcinomas are quite common in the lower leg and their appearance is often not typical. If an ulcer does not heal when properly treated, a biopsy of the ulcer edge should be taken. This can be done very simply using local anaesthetic. Vasculitic ulcers which occur in patients with auto immune disease also commonly occur in this region, probably because the skin of the lower leg has a relatively poorer blood supply than skin elsewhere. Arterial ulcers are usually seen on the foot. The are painful and usually have a punched out appearance. Arterial insufficiency, however, may compound the problem of a venous ulcer and make healing more difficult.

There are also other rarer causes of ulceration.

Management

Venous ulcers are the result of defective venous return. If the venous return is restored the ulcer will heal. One way to restore the venous return is to put the patient into a hospital bed with the feet elevated above heart level and the ulcer will heal. This treatment is frequently undertaken but it is very expensive in terms of hospital beds and lost earnings by the patient. In older patients prolonged bedrest is a positive threat to life.

A better way from everybody's point of view is to treat the patient as an outpatient, improving venous return by restoring the efficiency of the calf muscle pump. This is done by compressing the calf in an elastic stocking. The compression needs to be strong enough to overcome the hydrostatic pressure within the veins and needs to be graduated so that it is stronger at the bottom than at the top. The patient is instructed to go for regular, brisk walks. The calf muscles pump the blood out of the leg in the normal way and the stocking prevents it refluxing between muscle contractions, thus acting as an external valve. The stockings need to be worn from the moment the patient arises in the morning until the moment of getting into bed at night. Unless the underlying problem can be elimiated by operation (i.e. simple varicose veins), the patient must wear elastic stockings for life to prevent further ulceration.

Dressings are a social service to collect exudate. They have no therapautic affect but may be harmful by causing allergy. They should therefore be as simple (and as cheap) as possible.

Topical antibiotics should never be used. At best they can only sterilise slough. If living tissues are infected they need systemic antibiotics and they usually need to be used for several weeks for it is difficult to clear up cellulitis in poorly vascularised tissues.

Topical steroids may be used on allergic dermatitis and occasionally, with caution on the skin surrounding a vasculitic ulcer. They should never be applied to the ulcer itself and when they are used their use should be reviewed after one week at the very latest for they can make matters worse.

VARICOSE VEINS

Pathology

Varicose veins are either primary or secondary. *Primary varicose veins*, which are the vast majority, occur for no obvious reason. They tend to be familial and are much commoner in women than in men. They tend to appear first during times of hormonal change, i.e. at puberty (both sexes), during pregnancy and sometimes at the menopause. The symptoms are often exacerbated by oestrogenic contraceptives and by menstruation. There is clearly therefore a strong hormonal influence on them.

In young people usually the only demonstrable lesion is incompetence of the saphenous veins by the resulting increased venous pressure. This pressure is transmitted to the tributaries of the long saphenous vein which being thinner walled and lying more superficially than the saphenous vein, bear the brunt of the venous pressure increase. They dilate and lengthen. In 10-15% of patients the short saphenous vein is incompetent, sometimes in company with the long saphenous and sometimes alone.

In older patients there is a greater incidence of incompetent perforating veins and also of dilatation of the deep system. Since these occur more commonly in older patients it is reasonable to speculate that these changes are secondary to the superficial incompetence seen in younger patients. A possible mechanism for this is as follows:

> Blood pumped up the leg by the calf muscle pump refluxes down the long (or short) saphenous vein and is returned via the perforating veins to the deep system.
>
> This results in an increased volume of venous blood in the leg which will continue to increase as the superficial veins dilate.
>
> The flow through the perforators into the deep system will also increase. To accomodate this extra blood flow the perforating and deep veins will dilate thus eventually making their valves incompetent.

Perforator and deep vein incompetence may therefore result from primary varicose veins. This incompetence can be reversed. Treatment with an elastic stocking, with or without operating on the varicose veins will often restore the perforator and deep veins to normal. However, in many cases the changes appear to be irreversible. Early treatment of varicose veins is therefore desirable.

Secondary varicose veins are the result of thrombosis of the deep veins causing an increase in pressure in the deep system and reversal of the normal flow. Blood flows from the deep to the superficial system rather than the other way. This spoils the muscle pump and blood collects in the veins of the leg. The increase in pressure and blood volume produces dilatation and incompetence of the superficial system causing varicose veins. There is no point in operating on these varicose veins for the underlying problem remains. Sometimes, indeed, the superficial veins may be the main means of venous return from the limb and operating on these will make things much worse.

Diagnosis

Symptoms
The commonest symptom (about 85%) is aching of the leg which gets worse as the day goes on. Throbbing in the veins occurs with the same frequency. Cramp at night is a common symptom (50%). Patients do not associate this with varicose veins so it must be asked about directly. Swelling of the ankles and feet occurs in about 30%. Less than 10% get an ache in the groin but this is an important symptom which may lead to a wrong diagnosis. A presentation seen sometimes is a swelling in the groin which aches and is referred to the surgeon as a femoral hernia but is in fact an aching saphena varix (see below).

A family history is sought. If there is no family history in a male patient one is very suspicious that these are secondary varicose veins even though there may be no history suggestive of D.V.T. A history of D.V.T. is carefully taken. Superficial thrombosis is common in varicose veins patients so any history of thrombosis must be carefully evaluated. If the patient has had a lower limb fracture or joint replacement, the chances that there was a D.V.T. is over 70%.

Vulval varicosities may be the main source of filling of varicose veins and should always be asked about. A history of oral contraceptive use should also be asked for.

Physical Signs
Firstly the whole of the lower limb from groin to toes is examined with the patient standing. Venous dilatation in the groin (saphena varix) is felt for and a cough impulse elicited. In 20% of patients with sapheno femoral incompetence this will be absent for there will be a valve in the external iliac vein. The distribution of the veins is noted. The suprapubic and lower abdominal areas are examined for venous collaterals, indicating previous unilateral or bilateral ilio femoral thrombosis. The patient is turned around and the upper end of the short saphenous vein is palpated. To do this the patient is asked to stand on the contralateral limb and relax the muscles

bounding the popliteal fossa by allowing the knee on the side to be examined to flex a little. If the short saphenous vein is of normal calibre or impalpable it is not incompetent. If it feels dilated its position is marked on the skin with a pen.

It is important to look for vulval varicosities running from the vulva down the medial side of the upper thigh.

The patient then lies on the couch with the leg raised and the blood is stroked out of the veins. A 1 cm rubber tube is then fixed tightly around the top of the thigh using an artery forceps to secure it. This tourniquet must be tight enough to move the skin inwards for a distance greater than the diameter of the saphenous vein which may be 2 cm or so wide. Fat will tend to move from under the tourniquet so allowance must be made for this. In a very fat thigh it may be impossible to get the tourniquet tight enough to occlude the saphenous vein.

The patient then stands up. If the veins remain empty for 15 seconds it implies that the veins fill from above the tourniquet and are therefore filling from the sapheno femoral junction or the vulva (or both). If there is evidence of vulval varicosities, while the high tourniquet is on, pressure should be put over the external inguinal ring with one thumb and over the femoral ring with the other. The tourniquet is released by an assistant and the problem is assessed by removing first one thumb and then the other.

If a high tourniquet does not control the varicose veins, they must be filling from below the tourniquet. The tourniquet is applied just above the knee. If this controls the veins, a thigh perforating vein is incompetent. If control is still poor a tourniquet is put on the thigh and another just below the upper end of the short saphenous. The latter is firmly compressed with a thumb and the lower tourniquet released. If the thumb controls the varicosities and they fill again after removal of the thumb, short saphenous incompetence is present. If the tourniquet below the knee does not control the varicosities it means there are incompetent perforating veins in the calf. The exact position of these does not matter. They will be associated with venous blowouts which will be dealt with by operation or injection. Using the tourniquets may sound complicated but in fact it is only the thoughtful application of simple hydrodynamics and could be worked out by anybody. The important message here is that the tourniquet should be applied tightly enough. Failure to do this is very common.

Investigation

If there is ever any suspicion of a previous deep vein thrombosis a venogram is done.

Operation or injection is contraindicated after D.V.T. Venography is also often useful where diagnosis is not straight forward and one is not sure clinically where the veins are filling from.

Treatment

Female patients should stop all oestrogen intake for at least one month before operation because of the increased danger of D.V.T.

The incompetence needs to be dealt with by ligation. This most often means saphenofemoral ligation or short sapheno/popliteal ligation. Vulval varicosities are best ligated at the external inguinal ring. In early varicose veins the varicosities will slowly disappear, taking up to one year to get a perfect symptomatic and cosmetic result. In over 90% of men and 50% of women simple ligation will give a perfect symptomatic result. A good cosmetic result can be obtained either by avulsing the residual varices through tiny incisions or by injection and compression. The former is quick for the patient but slow and tedious for the surgeon, whereas the latter is quick for the surgeon but tedious for the patient whose legs must be compressed for six weeks and who may need more than one session of injections. The end results are the same.

Secondary varicose veins should never be operated on. It will do no good. They should be treated with elastic stockings. Primary varicose veins can also be treated satisfactorily with elastic stockings if operation is contraindicated for medical reasons or refused.

Elastic stockings can also be used as a diagnostic test to see if symptoms are due to varicose veins or some other problem. They will cure varicose veins symptoms but not symptoms due to other conditions.

In summary, it is important to work out the anatomy of varicose veins before prescribing any form of treatment for them. It is not necessary to remove the long saphenous vein for it is the tributaries which are varicosed and the long saphenous vein is a useful spare part. It is important to recognise which patients have incurable varicose veins and not to operate on these. It is important to realise that injections work very well provided the underlying long, short or vulval vein incompetence is dealt with and that injections alone should only be used to treat specific varicosities which have bled or are in danger of bleeding. If there is any doubt as to whether or not symptoms are due to varicose veins, use of an elastic stocking for a week or two helps with the diagnosis.

FURTHER READING FOR INTEREST

Way, L.W.: Current Surgical Diagnosis and Management. 8th Edition, 1988 . Appleton and Lange. Pp 715-737

FURTHER READING FOR FINALS

NIL

NOTES

Tutorial 14

Common Skin Malignancies

INTRODUCTION

In our country approximately 10,000 new patients with malignant skin tumours present each year, 800 of whom have primary malignant melanomas. At least 50% of all these tumours are basal cell carcinomas and two thirds of these arise on the head and neck.

There has been a dramatic increase in the incidence of all cutaneous malignancy in recent years.

Skin malignancy is rare in Maoris and Polynesians and melanoma is exceptional.

There are three common skin tumours which can be distinguished clinically according to the table

TABLE 1

Diagnostic Features of the Three Common Tumours

Tumour	History	Symptoms	Appearance
Basal Cell Carcinoma	Often 1 year or more	Often none	Local pearly nodule with surface blood vessels or diffuse spreading
Squamous Cell Carcinoma	Many months	Sometimes pain from secondary infection	Raised edge, often symmetrical, with central keratin production
Malignant Melanoma	Few Months or Weeks	Irritation, Bleeding	Irregular border and surface contour; Irregular pigmentation; ulceration; rarely satellite nodules of tumour

BASAL CELL CARCINOMA

Old name was "Rodent Ulcer" but few patients now present with large areas of skin and bone erosion from this infiltrative type of lesion. Multiple tumours are frequent but metastases are very rare.

Treatment

Because of the potential of these tumours to cause such destruction all should be treated. Surgical excision, usually on the basis of clinical appearance, with a margin of 0.5cm is sufficient.

Recurrences occur in 50% if histology shows tumour at the excision margins. If there has been complete excision, recurrence is only 5%

SQUAMOUS CELL CARCINOMA

The key to diagnosis is the presence of surface keratin. This together with the features shown in the table indicate the likelihood that the lesion is a squamous cell carcinoma.

The lesions metastasize to lymph nodes and more widely if not treated. It is rare for a tumour less than 0.5 cm in diameter to metastasize.

Treatment

The tumour is excised with a 1 cm margin of normal skin. Surgical elimination of multiple low grade squamous cell carcinomas or premalignant keratoses of the face and scalp is often impractical in the elderly patient. The daily application of the cytoxic 5% 5-Fluoro-uracil cream over a 2 week period can be used instead.

Note:

A benign *kerato acanthoma* is a rapidly growing skin lesion which resolves spontaneously after a few months. Since these lesions are very similar in appearance to squamous cell carcinomas, most surgeons advise excision.

MALIGNANT MELANOMA

Introduction

The most potentially dangerous skin cancer is malignant melanoma. It arises from melanocytes in the basal layers of the epidermis. The incidence of melanoma worldwide is steadily increasing, the highest incidence being in Australasia. There are three common types of melanoma.

Clinical and Histological Classification

Lentigo Maligna Melanoma

This is the least common and the least malignant. It is a slow growing, flat brown lesion with blotchy pigmentation and the outline is very irregular. It is seen most often in older patients on the temple or malar region where it is called 'Hutchinson's freckle' after Sir Jonathan Hutchinson (1828-1913), the famous London surgeon. Malignant change can be detected by the formation of darker areas and nodules or a general thickening.

Superficial Spreading Melanoma

This is the most common type and may occur on any part of the body. It is a slightly elevated and perhaps crusty brown lesion with an irregular but well defined edge.

Nodular Melanoma

This is not as common as superficial spreading melanoma but, being thicker, is more malignant. It is usually a uniform shade of grey, black or blue with a convex raised shape that can be felt. It may have a smooth surface and sharp edge and may be ulcerated.

In 1981 Dr A Breslow showed the relationship between thickness of the melanoma and recurrence or metastases (Table 2)

TABLE 2

Thickness (mm)	Percentage with recurrence or Metastases at 5 years
< .76	0%
0.76 - 1.5	33%
1.51 - 2.25	32%
2.26 - 3	69%
> 3	84%

It is now realised that the clinical descriptions of superficial spreading and nodular melanomas do not have prognostic value but the advent of measurement of the thickness of malignant melanoma has shown that thickness for thickness there is no difference in prognosis.

Differential Diagnosis

The appearance of a new pigmented naevus should arouse suspicion of melanoma. Pigmented skin lesions include *junctional naevi, dysplastic naevi, pigmented basal cell carcinomas, seborrhoeic keratosis* and *blue naevi*.

Treatment

All agree that excision of the presenting lesion is the correct initial therapy for the histological proven melanoma. Other aspects of management are vigorously debated.

Definitive treatment must be modified depending upon the type and location of the melanoma, the depth of invasion and the presence of lymph node involvement. The risk of local recurrence depends more on the thickness of the lesion than the width of the surgical margin. One to two cm margins for thin lesions and three cm margins for thick lesions (>1mm) are advocated by most authorities. If the regional lymph nodes are involved and there are no signs of distant metastases a node dissection is performed. Some surgeons also perform prophylactic node dissections for thick lesions.

About 30-40% of patients with malignant melanoma will eventually die from metastatic disease.

FURTHER READING FOR INTEREST

Emmet, A (1988): The Bare Facts. The Effect of Sun on the Skin. Williams and Wilkins and Associates Ltd.,Sydney

Cushieri, A. et al.: Essential Surgical Practice. 2nd Edition. Wright, London. Pp 225-259

FURTHER READING FOR FINALS

Nil

NOTES

INDEX

Abdomen
    acute 24–32
    history in 24–25
    physical examination in 25
    trauma to 82
    wall of
        hernias of 76–79
Abscess 9, 28
Acidosis
    metabolic 17
    respiratory 17
ACTH 6
Adenitis, cervical 64
Adenoid cystic carcinoma, of parotid gland 63
Adenomas
    colorectum 54–55, 56
    thyroid 61
Age, and surgical risk 2
Airway
    in basic life support 83
Albumin, serum, 2
Aldosterone 6
Alert state of consciousness, defined 84
Alkaline phosphatase
    in hepatobiliary disorders 38, 39
Alkalosis
    metabolic 17
    respiratory 17
Amino Acids
    in parenteral nutrition 20
Anal Canal. See also Anorectum, Anus, and Rectum
    anatomy of 51
Anal Fissure 53
Analgesia 7
Anastomosis
    colon 57
    gastro-duodenal 47, 49
    gastro-jejunal 49
Anaemia
    from gastro-intestinal blood loss 44
Anaesthesia
    complications of 6
    management of, during operations 6
Aneurysms
    aortic, ruptured 31
    arterial 89
    atherosclerotic 89, 90

    extracranial carotid 89, 90–91
    femoral 93
    infrarenal abdominal aortic 92
    popliteal 93
Angiodysplasia 57
Angiography 90, 91, 93, 94
Angioplasty
    percutaneous 93
Anorectum
    anatomy of 57, 54
Antibiotics
    as prophylaxis for infection 3
Anticoagulants 10
Antidiuretic hormone 6
Antithyroid drugs 62
Antrectomy and Vagotomy 49
Anus. See also Anal Canal, Anorectum, and Rectum 51-54
Aortic Aneurysm
    infrarenal abdominal 31, 91
    ruptured 90–91
Aortoiliofemoral reconstruction 92, 93
Appendicectomy 26
Appendicitis 25
    acute 25–26
    pelvic 26
Artery
    aneurysm of 31, 89, 90, 93
    catheterization of, 91
    degenerative disease of 90
    distal, reconstruction of 92
    peripheral
        insufficiency of 92
        occlusion of 93, 94
Atelectasis
    postoperative 8

Barium enema 56
Basal cell carcinoma
    of skin 98, 106, 107
Battle's sign 85
Bicarbonate 15
Bile duct(s)
    obstruction of 35–42
    tumours of 36, 38
Biliary Colic 26, 37
Biliary Pancreatitis 38

Biliary Stricture 36, 38, 42
Bilirubin 35, 36
Billroth procedures 47, 49
Blood
    coagulation defects 21, 42
    occult, faecal 57
    passage of, per rectum 51–58
    transfusion of 8, 21
Blood glucose estimations
    during operations 3
Body composition 12–13
Body water 12, 13
Bowel. See Intestine
Bowel prep. 3
Brain
    injury to 84
Branchial cyst 63
Breast-female
    carcinoma of 67–74
        adjuvant chemotherapy 72–74
        advanced, treatment of 73–74
        biopsy in 67
        cytologic examination in 69
        drugs used in 72–74
        early detection of 69
        pathologic types of 68
        radiation therapy of 71
        radionuclide scanning in 70
        self-examination for 68
        staging of 70
    examination of 68–69
    reconstruction of 71
Breslow's classification of melanoma 108

Calculi
    salivary 62
    ureteric 31
Calories
    requirements of 19
Cancer. See specific types and organs
Carcinoma. See specific types
    unknown, primary 64–65
Cardiac disease
    and surgical patients 2, 3, 9-10
Cardiac failure
    postoperative 10
Cardiooesophageal sphincter, incompetent 80
Carotid endarterectomy 91
Catecholamines 6
Catheterization
    of bladder 21, 84

Charcot's triad 37, 38
Chemotherapy
    in breast cancer 73–74
    combination 73–74
    scientific basis of 72–73
Chest
    injuries to, traumatic 82, 83, 85
Cholangiography, percutaneous
transhepatic 40
Cholangiopancreatography, endoscopic
retrograde 40
Cholangitis 37-38
    sclerosing, biliary obstruction due to 36
Cholecystectomy 41
Cholecystitis
    acute 26-27, 37
Cholecystography 39
Choledocholithiasis 37–38, 41
Cholelithiasis 37–38, 41
Cholestasis 35
Claudication 92
Closure of wounds 9
Coagulation of blood 21, 42, 39
Coffee-ground vomitus 44
Colectomy, ileostomy after 58
Colic 35
    biliary 26, 37
    renal 31
Colitis
    Crohn's 57, 58
    ulcerative 57, 58
Collar-stud abscess 64
Colloids 7, 8, 21
Colon. See also Intestine(s), large 56–58
    carcinoma of 57
    preoperative preparation of 3
Colonoscopy
    fiberoptic 30, 56, 57
Colostomy 30, 55
Computerized tomography 28, 40, 85, 89
Consciousness
    level of, examination for 84
Consent, informed 1
Consultations, preoperative 1
Cortisol 6
Courvoisier's law 38
Crohn's Disease
    of large intestine 57–58

of small intestine 58
Critical care, department of 7, 21
CT scan
   in jaundice 40
   in trauma 85
Cystic hygroma 64
Cysts
   branchial 63
   thyroglossal 63
   thyroid 61

Deep vein thrombosis 1, 2, 4, 10, 101
Dehiscence of wound
   postoperative 9
Dehydration
   surgical 15
Diabetes
   and surgical patient 3, 89
Diaphragm
   hernia of 80
Diet(s)
   enteral 19, 20
   parenteral 19, 20
Diverticul(a)
   of colon 30, 57
   pharyngooesophageal 64
Diverticulitis, of colon 30–31, 57
Diverticulosis, of colon 57
Drains, percutaneous 26, 28, 31
Dukes staging system 55
Duodenum
   ulcer of 27, 44–47
Dysplastic nevi, and malignant melanoma 109

ECF depletion 15–16
Ectopic Pregnancy 31
Eldery patient, and surgical risk 2
Electrocardiogram, preoperative 1
Electrolyte(s)
   in body fluids 15
   depletion of 16–17
   disorders of 16–17
   and fluid volume disorders 15–17
   in gastric juice 15
   in gastrointestinal fluids 15
   management of 17–19
Electrolyte therapy, principles of 15–19
Embolism
   in atherosclerosis 89
   pulmonary 10, 22
Emergency room care 82–87

Emotional background of patients 1
Endoscopy 46
Epididymal cyst 78

Fat 12
Fever 8

Gallstones 36–38
   Cholesterol 36
   Pigment 36
Gas
   free, in acute abdomen 25, 27
   intestinal 25
Gastrectomy
   subtotal 49
   total 49
Gastric carcinoma 45, 48
Gastric juice 44
Gastric ulcer 44-47
Gastric strangulation 80
Gastritis 44
Gastroduodenoscopy 46
Gastrooesophageal sphincter 80
Gastrointestinal fluid losses 14, 15
Gastrointestinal haemorrhage, lower 51–58
Gastrointestinal motility, postoperative alterations to 7
Gastrointestinal tract
   lower, haemorrhage of 51–58
   postoperative care of 7
   preparation of for surgery 3
   upper, haemorrhage of 44–49
Glucagon 6
Glucose
   in parenteral nutrition 20
Glycogen 21
Goitre 61–62
   diffuse and multinodular 62
   simple 61
Grave's disease 62
Groin
   anatomy of 76
   hernias of 77–79
Growth hormone 6

H_2 receptor antagonists, in duodenal ulcer 46, 47
Hamartoma
   rectum 55
Hartmann procedure 30

Headache 14
Health assessment, general 1
Heart disease
    ischaemic 3
    valvular 3
Haemaccel 21
Haematemesis 44
Haemolytic jaundice 35
Haemoperitoneum 84
Haemorrhage
    from peptic ulcer 44–47
    gastrointestinal 51–58
        lower 51–58
        upper 44–49
Haemorrhoids
    degree 52
    external 53
    internal 52
    thrombosed 52
    treatment of 53
Haemothorax 83, 85
Helicobacter pylori 45,
Heparin 4, 10

Hernia(s) 76–80
    epigastric 79
    femoral 79
    of groin 76–79
    hiatal 80
    incarcerated (irreducible) 77
    inguinal
        operations for 78, 79
        sliding 77, 80
    paraoesophageal 80
    reducible 77
    Shouldice repair of 78, 79
    umbilical 79
Hiatal hernia
    para-oesophageal 80
    sliding 80
HIDA scan, of gallbladder 40
Hormone(s)
    response of, to surgery 6
Hutchinson's freckle 108
Hydrocele 77, 78
Hypertension
    portal 48
Hyperthyroidism 61, 62
Hypoalbuminaemia 2
Hypokalaemia 16, 17
Hyponatraemia 14, 16

Hypovolaemic shock 21
^{131}I 61, 62
ICF 13
Ileoanal anastomosis, with J Pouch 58
Ileostomy 58
Incarcerated (irreducible) hernia 77
Infarction, myocardial
    postoperative 9-10
Infection(s)
    of surgical wound 9
Inflammatory bowel disease 57–58
Inflammatory carcinoma of breast 69
Informed consent 1
Inguinal hernia 77-79
    direct 79
    indirect 78
    sliding 77
Inguinal rings, examination of, in small intestinal obstruction 29
Injured patient
    evaluation of 82–86
    management of 82–87
Inotropic agents 21
Insulin 3, 6
Interpleural block 7
Intestine(s)
    large
        anatomy of 56
        cancer of 57
        Crohn's disease of 58
        diverticular disease of 30
        colonoscopic examination of 57
        haemorrhage 56, 57
        lymphatic drainage of 56
        obstruction of 30
        polyps of 56
        preoperative preparation of 3
        x-ray examination of 56
        tumours of 30
        volvulus of 30
    obstruction of 30, 57
    small, see also Duodenum, Ileum and Jejunum
        Crohn's disease of 58
        obstruction of 29
Intracellular fluid 13
Intravenous solutions, composition of 17–18
Intravenous therapy 17-19
Intubation
    nasogastric 29

Jaundice 2, 35–42
Jejunostomy 49
Junctional nevi 109

Keratoses
  solar 107

Large intestine. See Intestine(s) large
Larynx 60
Lean body mass (LBM) 12
Lentigo maligna melanoma 108
Lithotripsy 41
Lung(s)
  injuries to 83, 85
Lymphatics
  of colon 56
  of head and neck 60
Lymphomas 64

Malignant melanoma 106, 107–109
Mallory-Weiss syndrome 48
Mammary dysplasia 67
Mammography 69
Mammoplasty 71
Mastectomy 68–69
Melanoma
  malignant 106, 107-109
  nodular 108
  superficial spreading 108
  staging of 108
Melaena 44
Metabolic acidosis 17
Metabolic alkalosis 17, 47
Metabolism, and nutrition 6-7, 12-20
Metastases
  neck 64–65
Molar KCI 7, 18, 19, 47
Mucoepidermoid carcinoma, of parotid gland 63
Mucosal resistance in stomach and duodenum 44, 45
Murphy's sign 27, 37
Myocardial infarction 21
  postoperative 9–10

Naevi
  junctional 109
Neck
  inflammatory masses of 64
  lymphatic anatomy of 60
  metastases in 64–65
Nerve(s)
  facial 61
  recurrent laryngeal 60
Nissen fundoplication 80
Nitrogen
  in parenteral nutrition 19
Normal saline 17, 18
Nutrition
  assessment of
    and surgical risk 2
  enteral 2, 19, 20
  parenteral 2, 19, 20
Nutritional pathophysiology 19
Nutritional requirements 19–20
Nutritional support
  complications of 20

Obesity
  and surgical risk 2
Obstipation in acute abdomen 78
Obstruction
  intestinal 29, 30
  posthepatic 35
Occlusion(s)
  of peripheral artery 92–93, 94
Oncogene 72
Opiates
  for postoperative pain 7

Pancreas
  adeno-carcinoma of 36
Pancreatectomy 42
Pancreatic abscess 28
  pseudocyst 28
Pancreaticoduedenectomy 42
Pancreatitis
  acute 28, 38
Paraoesophageal hernia 80
Paralysis, facial 61
Parathyroid glands 60
Parenteral nutrition
  complications of 20
Parietal cell vagotomy 27
Parotid gland 61, 62, 63
Pelvis
  fractures of 84, 85, 86
Peptic ulcer

haemorrhage 44, 46-47
perforated 27, 29
pyloric obstruction due to 45, 47
Percutaneous drainage 26, 28, 31
Perforation
　colonic diverticulum 57
　duodenal ulcer 27
　gallbladder 27
Peritoneum
　adhesions of 29
Peritonitis
　biliary 27, 37
　faecal 31
　in acute abdomen 25
Pharyngeal diverticulum 64
Plasma substitutes 7
Pneumonia
　postoperative 3, 9
Pneumothorax 83, 85
Polyps
　of colon and rectum 54
Polyposis 56
Popliteal artery
　aneurysms of 93
Portal Hypertension 48
Postoperative care 7–10
Postoperative period 7–10
　immediate 7–8
　intermediate 8–10
Postoperative wound infections 9
Potassium
　concentration of, disorders of 16-17
Preoperative anaesthetic evaluation 1–2
Preoperative care 1–5
Preoperative evaluation 1
Preoperative preparation 3–5
Proctitis 55
Procto-colitis 56
Protein-energy malnutrition 19
Protein
　requirements of 19–20
Pseudocyst, pancreatic 28
Pulmonary care, postoperative 8, 9
Pulmonary embolism 10, 21
Pulmonary function, preoperative evaluation
　of 1, 2, 3
Pyloric obstruction, due to peptic ulcer 45, 47
Pyloroplasty 47, 49

Radiation therapy
　for breast cancer 71
Radical-en-bloc mastectomy 70, 71
Radioactive iodine 61, 62
Rectum. See also Anal canal, Anorectum and Anus
　cancer of 55
　　classification 55
　　and colitis 57, 58
　polyps 54
　tumours of 55
Reflux oesophagitis 80
Respiratory acidosis 17
Respiratory alkalosis 17
Respiratory complications, postoperative 8, 9
Reticulosarcoma 64

Salivary Glands 62–63
Septic shock 21
Shock 20–22
S.P.P.S. 7, 8, 21
Squamous cell carcinoma
　of skin 98, 106, 107
Thromboembolism
　pulmonary 10
Thyroglossal duct 63
Thyroid gland
　anatomy 60
　cancer of 61–62
　nodules of, evaluation of 61–62
　tumours of
　　benign 61
　　malignant 61–62
Thyroid goitre 61–62
Thyroidectomy, subtotal 8, 61, 62
Thyroiditis 62
Thyrotoxicosis 61, 62
Total body potassium 13
Trace elements
　in parenteral nutrition 20
Transfusion(s) 21
Transhepatic cholangiography 40
Transient ischaemic attack 90, 91
Trauma 82–87
Tuberculosis
　of neck 64
Ulcers
　duodenal 44–47

gastric 44-47
peptic
    haemorrhage from 44, 46–47
    perforated 27, 28, 44
    pyloric obstruction due to 45, 47
venous 40

Ulcerative colitis 36, 57-58
Ultrasonography
    in acute abdomen 26, 27
    in arterial disease 89, 90, 94
    in gallbladder disease 40
Umbilical hernia
    paraumbilical 79
    infantile 79
Ureteric Stone 31
Urinary Retention 8

Vagotomy
    truncal 48–49
    parietal cell 27, 46, 48
Varices
    bleeding 48
Varicose veins 100–103
Vas deferens 76
Vein stripping 103
Veins
    varicose 4

Venography 10
Venous insufficiency 10
Venous pressure 97–98
Venous stasis, reduction of 99
Venous system
    anatomy of 97–98
    diseases of 97–103
    physiology of 97–98
Venous ulcers 97–99
Vitamin(s)
    in parenteral nutrition 20
Volume depletion 15
Volvulus, of sigmoid 30

Water, body 12, 13
Weight, body, loss of 2
Whipple procedure 42
Wound(s)
    complications of 9
    dehiscence of 9
    infection, prevention of 9
    postoperative care of 9
    surgical
        care of 9
        infection in 9

Yersinia 26